ETHNIC SKIN

MEDICAL AND SURGICAL

ETHNIC SKIN
MEDICAL AND SURGICAL

Bernett L. Johnson, Jr., MD
Professor and Vice Chairman
Department of Dermatology
University of Pennsylvania School of Medicine
Philadelphia, Pennsylvania

Ronald L. Moy, MD
Associate Clinical Professor
UCLA Division of Dermatology
Director of Dermatologic Surgery
VA West Los Angeles Medical Center
Editor in Chief, Dermatologic surgery
Los Angeles, California

Gary M. White, MD
Chief, Department of Dermatology
Kaiser Permanente, San Diego;
Assistant Clinical Professor
Department of Dermatology
University of California School of Medicine
San Diego, California

with 355 illustrations

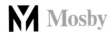 Mosby

St. Louis Baltimore Boston Carlsbad
Chicago Minneapolis New York Philadelphia Portland
London Milan Sydney Tokyo Toronto

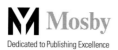

Mosby

Dedicated to Publishing Excellence

A Times Mirror Company

Executive Editor: Susie H. Baxter
Developmental Editor: Anne Gunter
Project Manager: Carol Sullivan Weis
Production Editor: Karen M. Rehwinkel
Designer: Jen Marmarinos
Manufacturing Manager: Karen Lewis

Printed in the United States of America
Composition and Lithography/color film by Top Graphics
Printing/binding by Walsworth Press, Inc.

Mosby, Inc.
11830 Westline Industrial Drive
St. Louis, Missouri 63146

Library of Congress Cataloging-in-Publication Data

Johnson, Bernett L.
    Ethnic skin : medical and surgical / Bernett L. Johnson, Jr.,
  Ronald L. Moy, Gary M. White.
       p.   cm.
    Includes bibliographical references and index.
    ISBN 0-8151-5687-1
    1. Skin—Diseases.   2. Ethnic groups—Diseases.   3. Skin—Surgery.
  4. Ethnic groups—Health and hygiene.   5. Human skin color.
  I. Moy, Ronald L.   II. White, Gary M., 1961-   . III. Title.
    [DNLM: 1. Skin Diseases—ethnology.   2. Skin Diseases—therapy.
  3. Ethnic Groups.   4. Asian Americans.   5. Blacks.   6. Hispanic
  Americans.   WR 140 J66e 1998]
  RL73.3.J64   1998
  616.5—dc21
  DNLM/DLC
  for Library of Congress   97-45884
                                                                 CIP

98 99 00 01 02 / 9 8 7 6 5 4 3 2 1

To my family, Mary-Martha, Susanne, Logan, Brian, *and* Keith,
and to my mentors for their support, wisdom, and counsel.

Bernett L. Johnson, Jr.

To my wife, Lisa, *my children*, Lauren and Erin, *and my parents*,
Howard *and* Jenny, *for all their love and support.*

Ronald L. Moy

To Jolly *and* Herman, *my wonderful mom and dad.*

Gary M. White

Contributors

Amy J. McMichael, MD
Assistant Professor of Dermatology,
Bowman Gray School of Medicine,
Wake Forest University,
Winston-Salem, North Carolina

Vic A. Narurkar, MD
Assistant Professor of Clinical Dermatology,
Department of Dermatology,
University of California School of Medicine, Davis,
Sacramento, California

Larry Seifert, MD
Assistant Clinical Professor,
Division of Plastic Surgery,
University of California School of Medicine, Los Angeles,
Los Angeles, California

Daniel P. Taheri, MD
UCLA Division of Dermatology,
University of California School of Medicine, Los Angeles,
Los Angeles, California

Preface

An individual's ethnic background can and does modify the presentation and severity of disease. Ethnicity can also modify the patient's response to a treatment regimen just on the basis of the individual's inherited characteristics. This is especially true in skin disease. Diagnosing and recognizing skin disorders in individuals whose skin color is not white requires an understanding of how ethnicity modifies disease and how treatment should be tailored to be most effective in various ethnic groups.

This book provides a practical look at dermatologic disease in patients of different ethnic groups (black, Asian, and Hispanic) and tries to point out the effect of ethnicity on dermatologic disease. The surgical aspects of the treatment of dermatologic disease in diverse ethnic groups and the sequelae of this treatment (pigmentary and fibroblastic changes) are included in this text; this is an area that is rarely covered in other texts that discuss the treatment of skin diseases. Also in this text, there is particular emphasis on results expected after surgical procedures, regardless of whether they are performed for therapeutic or cosmetic reasons. We have also made an effort throughout the text to highlight important points that provide brief but important take-home messages for the reader.

Bernett L. Johnson, Jr.
Ronald L. Moy
Gary M. White

Contents

ETHNIC SKIN

MEDICAL AND SURGICAL

General Considerations

Differences in Skin Type

Bernett L. Johnson, Jr.

Ethnic skin dermatoses are those that occur in people of different ethnic backgrounds (i.e., black, white, Asian, and Hispanic) and are modified or influenced by the characteristic differences in ethnic skin, such as pigment; follicular response; curved, flat hair; and fibroblast reactivity.

PIGMENT

Black skin has more pigment than other ethnic skin types. Melanin pigment is produced in melanocytes, the number and distribution of which are the same for black and nonblack skin. The difference in color is due to greater melanocyte function in black skin related to the production of larger and more melanized melanosomes (stages three and four). Because black skin has more melanin, the effect on melanin pigment by dermatologic disease or environmental factors is heightened. This increased effect becomes the basis for the dermatologic changes of hyperpigmentation and hypopigmentation.

Melanin pigment is produced in melanocytes, the number and distribution of which are the same for black and nonblack skin. The difference in color is due to greater melanocyte function in black skin related to the production of larger and more melanized melanosomes (stages three and four).

FOLLICULAR RESPONSE

Follicular responsiveness, or reactivity, is seen clinically in the follicular accentuation common to many dermatologic diseases in black skin. For example, follicular accentuation can be seen in pityriasis rosea, atopic dermatitis, nummular eczema, and sarcoidosis.

FIBROBLAST

Fibroblast hyperresponsivity, thought to be induced by mast cell/fibroblast interaction and prolonged by a decrease in collagenase activity, leads to keloid formation, which is another characteristic of black skin.

CURLY HAIR

The hair in black skin is flattened and found in a follicle that is set at an acute angle in the skin (Figure 1-1). These anatomic findings lead to hair that curls acutely. This characteristic causes the clinical findings in pseudofolliculitis barbae and acne keloidalis. Curly hair also tends to spontaneously knot and fracture. Curling black hair is the "root" cause of many dermatologic problems in black women. Cultural concepts on the beauty of hair and its management lead to many of the problems seen in the scalps and hair of black women, for whom style dictates straight hair. The process of producing straight hair with either chemicals (processing) or heat and oils (hot comb technique) causes hair fracture, scalp scarring, and temporary or permanent alopecia.

ASHINESS

People who have dark skin become "ashy" white when their skin is dry and scaly. This same scaling occurs in nonblack skin but is clinically inapparent. Because the "ashy" color is considered unacceptable by some, many blacks use oils and/or petrolatum to mask it. This in turn leads to oil folliculitis and appears to adversely affect acne.

These factors, plus those dermatoses that manifest differently in black skin, are presented in greater depth in the chapters that follow.

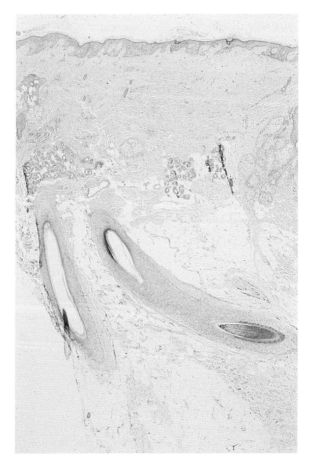

Figure 1-1   Hair follicles set at an acute angle in black scalp skin. (×20.)

Histologic Differences

Bernett L. Johnson, Jr.

BLACK SKIN

Black skin does have distinct histologic features, the most significant of which is pigmentation (Figures 2-1 and 2-2). Pigment in normal black skin is always present at the basal cell layer and may occur in granular form several layers higher in the epidermis. The stratum corneum may also be pigmented, a feature not seen in nonblack skin unless a tumor is present.

Although there is an increase in pigmentation histologically in black skin, the number of melanocytes/mm^2 of tissue is the same in black skin as in nonblack skin.[1] The difference in color seen externally and on histologic sections is a reflection of pigment granule (melanosome) production, size, and dispersion, and the grouping of melanosomes in lysosomes. In black skin, melanosome production is greater, the melanosomes are larger, and they are dispersed instead of being packaged in lysosomal vacuoles.

The stratum corneum and epidermis in black skin tend to be thicker, although this is not an absolute finding. Inflammation in black skin most commonly produces hyperpigmentation; there is increased production of melanosomes associated with pigment dropping into the dermis from the disrupted basal cell and collecting in melanophages. Hypopigmentation may also occur but appears to be a less common finding after inflammatory insults. Solar elastosis, a common finding in nonblack skin, does occur in black skin, but it is less severe and develops at a later age. Follicular abnormalities are more common in black skin. The hair follicle lies at an acute angle to the surface, and follicular rupture occurs secondary to penetration of the follicle by a flattened, curled hair. This leads to inflammation and subsequent fibrosis (keloid) and is clinically expressed as pseudofolliculitis barbae and acne keloidalis. Chronic rubbing and/or scratching of black skin produces follicular hypertrophy, epidermal thickening (acanthosis), and greater pigmentation than is seen for the same amount of trauma in nonblack skin.

NONBLACK SKIN

Histologically, nonblack skin has less melanin on routine sections (Figure 2-3). In white skin, no melanin is appreciated in the basal cell layer. Follicular structures are vertically oriented and not curved, and the hair is oval to round. The stratum corneum and epidermis, by comparison, are thinner than in black skin. Pigment is increased in Asian and some Hispanic skin compared with white skin. Hispanic skin can show a great variation in pigmentation in the basal cell layer. Although the follicle is straight and perpendicular to the skin surface in Hispanics, the hair can vary from oval to flattened.

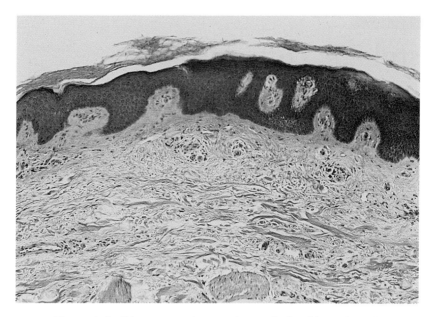

Figure 2-1　Linear, even pigmentation at the basal layer. (×20.)

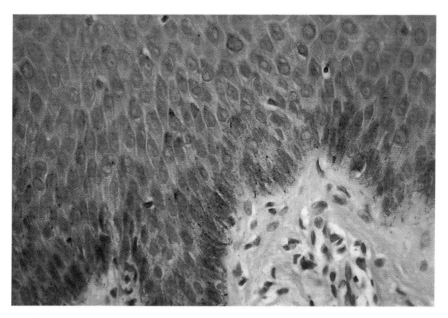

Figure 2-2　High magnification showing melanin granules (melanosomes) in basal and mid-spinus keratinocytes. (×400.)

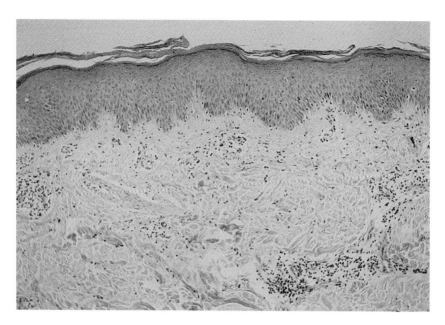

Figure 2-3   White skin without pigment at the basal cell layer. (×40.)

The follicular structures in Asian skin are not curved, and the hair is round. Pigmentation can be observed in the basal layer. Other than these differences, the histologic features of all skin types are similar when sites are matched.

REFERENCE

1. Staricco RJ, Pinkus H: Quantitative and qualitative data on the pigment cell of adult human epidermis, *J Invest Dermatol* 28:33, 1957.

Chapter 3

Skin Cancer

Daniel P. Taheri, Vic Narurkar, and Ronald L. Moy

Skin cancer is the most common type of malignancy in the United States[1,2]; however, the incidence of skin cancer in the darker-skinned population reportedly remains relatively low.[1-3] This has been attributed to increased pigmentation and melanosomal dispersion, which helps to protect against the ultraviolet (UV) rays of the sun, the most common cause of skin cancer.[4] For instance, the epidermis of blacks has a natural sun protection factor of approximately 13.[5] As a result of this protection, the skin cancer rate is much smaller in the more pigmented racial groups. However, with increased trends toward outdoor recreational activities and the depletion of the stratospheric ozone layer, an increased skin cancer rate among the various racial groups would be expected. Blacks have a higher morbidity and mortality rate as a result of skin cancer than their white counterparts. This difference is most likely related to the more advanced stage of disease at the time of presentation.[6]

Certain forms of skin cancer are more prevalent among the various ethnic groups. As with whites, basal cell carcinoma, squamous cell carcinoma, and malignant melanoma are the most common skin cancers occurring in blacks. Other malignancies include Bowen's disease, Kaposi's sarcoma, cutaneous T-cell lymphoma, and dermatofibrosarcoma protuberans.

BASAL CELL CARCINOMA

Basal cell carcinoma (BCC) is the most common cutaneous malignancy in whites. It occurs less commonly in blacks because the darker skin pigmentation plays a protective role against UVB radiation, the spectrum thought to be causative in the development of skin cancer[7,8] (Figure 3-1). The degree of pigmentation is also of importance. In one study, it was noted that blacks with lighter skin tones were more likely to be afflicted with skin cancer.[1] Other risk factors for BCC include prior radiation exposure, trauma, arsenic ingestion, nevus sebaceous, immunosuppression, and basal cell nevus syndrome.[9]

The major etiologic factor in BCC appears to be the intensity and duration of skin exposure to ultraviolet light. A majority of darker-skinned individuals who have been treated for skin cancers had excessive amounts of sun exposure during their youth. The degree of skin pigmentation also affects the frequency of BCC, with lighter-toned individuals more susceptible. BCC tends to present later in life, with the majority of patients being more than 50 years old.[1-3,7,10] Skin cancer also tends to be more prevalent among black females than males.[2,6,11] The anatomic distribution is similar among the two populations.[1,12] It has also been demonstrated that blacks and whites have a similar risk of developing BCC in non–sun-exposed skin.[13]

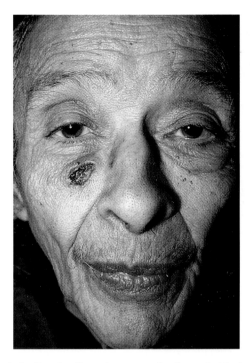

Figure 3-1 Basal cell carcinoma on the face of a black patient.

BCC in blacks and Asians is almost always of the pigmented type[1,3] and may be mistaken for malignant melanoma, seborrheic keratoses, or nevus sebaceous[3] (Figures 3-2 to 3-6). As for the specific subtype, one series reported 53% of BCCs in blacks to be of the solid or nodular histologic subtype, 44% of the combined solid and adenoid type, and 2% of the superficial type.[7]

The major etiologic factor in BCC appears to be the intensity and duration of skin exposure to ultraviolet light.

BCC in blacks and Asians is almost always of the pigmented type.

SQUAMOUS CELL CARCINOMA

Squamous cell carcinoma (SCC) is the most common skin cancer in blacks.[1,3] One study found 65% of SCC in blacks to involve non–sun-exposed areas, including the legs.[1] The opposite is found with whites, where the majority of SCCs are found in chronically sun-exposed skin. There is a higher mortality associated with SCC in blacks. A delay in the diagnosis and treatment in conjunction with a more aggressive nature of the tumor may account for this.

One study found 65% of SCC in blacks to involve non–sun-exposed areas.

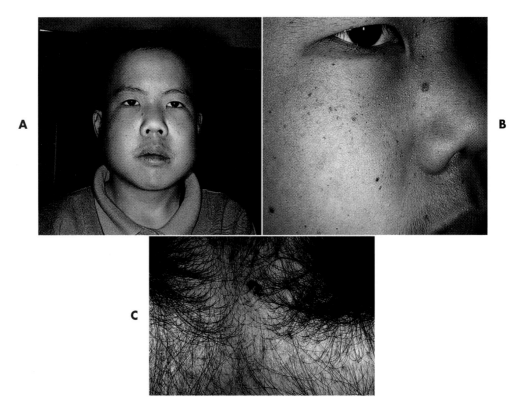

Figure 3-2   Basal cell nevus syndrome in an Asian child. This syndrome is an inherited disorder in which patients are prone to develop multiple basal cell carcinomas at an early age.

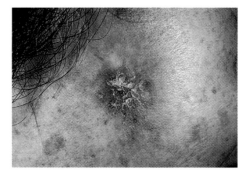

Figure 3-3   Basal cell carcinoma in an Asian male.

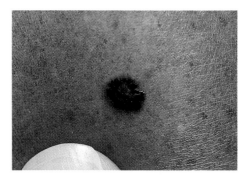

Figure 3-4   Pigmented basal cell carcinoma in a man from the Philippines.

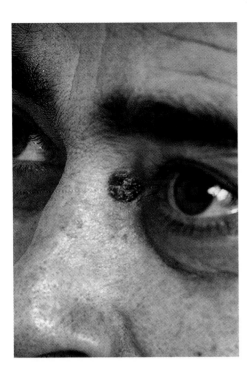

Figure 3-5 Pigmented basal cell carcinoma in a Hispanic patient.

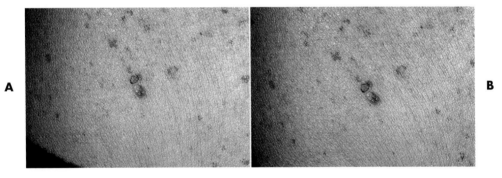

A   B

Figure 3-6 An example of xeroderma pigmentation, a genetic disorder in which patients are prone to develop multiple skin cancers at an early age.

Predisposing factors important in the development of SCC include scars from thermal and chemical burns, chronic inflammation, chronic leg ulcers, previous sites of irradiation, chemical carcinogens, albinism, and chronic discoid lupus erythematosus (DLE).[1,14] In Asians, SCC has also been associated with arsenic exposure.

The clinical presentation of SCC may vary. Differential diagnoses include psoriasis, eczema, infection, and trauma.[1] Biopsies should be performed on all nonhealing, persistent skin ulcers, regardless of the patient's ethnic origin.[6]

MALIGNANT MELANOMA

From 1987 to 1988, the annual rate of malignant melanoma in the United States for blacks was 0.9 per 100,000, whereas an incidence of 10.9 per 100,000 was reported for whites during the same period.[15] In the ethnic groups (blacks, Asians, and Native Americans), the majority of melanomas were found in non–sun-exposed skin, especially in the periungual, palmar, and plantar surfaces[16] (Figure 3-7). There is also a disproportionate number of the acral lentiginous type of melanoma in this population (Figures 3-8 to 3-10). Although blacks who get melanoma usually develop the acral lentiginous form, no significant difference was found in the incidence of plantar melanoma between blacks and whites.[17]

The majority of melanomas were found in non–sun-exposed skin, especially in the periungual, palmar, and plantar surfaces.

Acral lentiginous melanoma of the plantar type may be mistaken for a plantar wart. A histologic examination may be needed to differentiate between the two. A rare fungal infection called *tinea nigra palmaris* is also a differential diagnosis. This condition can be readily diagnosed when potassium hydroxide (KOH) scraping reveals fungal hyphae. The vertical growth phase in this type of melanoma can be deceptive, showing only a small degree of papular elevation associated with a deep invasion. Acral lentiginous melanoma has a fairly poor prognosis, with a 5-year survival rate of less than 50%.

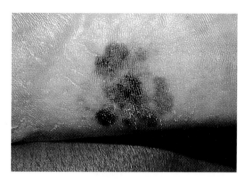

Figure 3-7   Melanoma on the sole of a black patient.

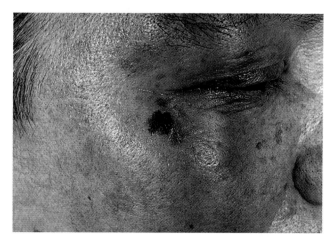

Figure 3-8   Lentigo malignant melanoma in a Hispanic patient.

CUTANEOUS T-CELL LYMPHOMA

Cutaneous T-cell lymphoma (CTCL) (See Figure 7-28) is a disease more commonly found in blacks,[18] with greater than twofold prevalence reported.[19] The etiology of CTCL remains unknown, although viruses and industrial exposures have been proposed as possible etiologic agents in the pathogenesis of this disease. Controlled studies have not been able to confirm a correlation.[18]

DERMATOFIBROSARCOMA PROTUBERANS

Dermatofibrosarcoma protuberans (DFSP) is a rare skin cancer that is thought to occur more frequently in blacks than in whites.[20] DFSP may clinically resemble a keloid, and therefore all suspicious lesions with an unusual appearance, such as those occurring in nontraumatized areas or those with rapid clinical growth, should undergo biopsy.[6]

DFSP may clinically resemble a keloid.

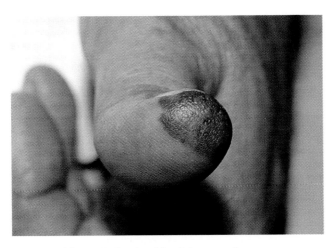

Figure 3-9   Acral lentiginous melanoma.

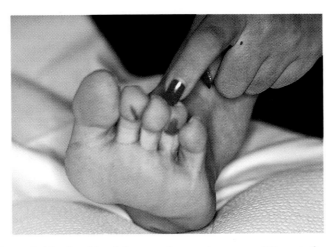

Figure 3-10   Acral lentiginous melanoma in a young Hispanic female.

KAPOSI'S SARCOMA

Kaposi's sarcoma is a skin cancer most commonly present in patients with AIDS. Blacks who have this type of skin cancer have shown a greater morbidity than patients of other ethnic backgrounds.[21] Kaposi's sarcoma also tends to progress at a faster pace for blacks with AIDS.[21,22]

BOWEN'S DISEASE

Bowen's disease in blacks or Asians presents clinically as a nonspecific scaling, hyperkeratotic, pigmented lesion.[1] Bowen's disease rarely shows pigmentation outside of the groin area in whites, but in blacks or Asians pigmentation is frequently seen in nongenital lesions.[23] Bowen's disease affects black women at a rate twice that of black men and most commonly affects covered skin.[24]

SUMMARY

A heightened awareness of skin cancer in the darkly-pigmented population is needed. Because of greater exposure to solar UV radiation, a continually increased incidence of skin cancer in this population is being witnessed. The early diagnosis and treatment of all suspicious lesions should be emphasized.

REFERENCES

1. Halder RM, Bang KM: Skin cancer in African Americans in the US, *Dermatol Clin* 6(3):397-407, 1988.
2. Mora RG, Burris R: Cancer of the skin in African Americans: a review of 128 patients with basal cell carcinoma, *Cancer* 47:1436-1438, 1981.
3. Altman A et al: Basal cell epithelioma in African-American patients, *J Am Acad Dermatol* 17:741-745, 1987.
4. Serna MJ, Vasquez FJ, Quintanilla E: Basal cell carcinoma in North American blacks, *J Am Acad Dermatol* 27:787-788, 1992.
5. Montagna W, Prota G, Kenney JA Jr: *Black skin structure and function*, London, 1993, Academic Press, pp 55-60.
6. Halder RM, Bridgeman-Shah S: Skin cancer in African Americans, *Cancer* 75:667-673, 1995.
7. Abreo F, Sanusi ID: Basal cell carcinoma in North American blacks, *J Am Acad Dermatol* 25(6):1005-1011, 1991.
8. Preston DS, Stern RS: Nonmelanoma cancers of skin, *N Engl J Med* 327:1649-1662, 1992.
9. Nguyen A, Whitaker DC, Frodel J: Differentiation of basal cell carcinoma, *Otolaryngol Clin North Am* 26:37-56, 1993.
10. Chorun L, Norris JE, Gupta M: Basal cell carcinoma in blacks: a report of 15 cases, *Ann Plast Surg* 33(1):90-95, 1994.
11. Matsuoka Ly, Schauer PK, Sordillo PP: Basal cell carcinoma in African-American patients, *J Am Acad Dermatol* 4:670-672, 1981.
12. Mora RG: Surgical and aesthetic considerations of cancer of the skin in the African American, *J Dermatol Surg Oncol* 12:24-31, 1986.
13. Schrek R: Cutaneous carcinoma: analysis of 20 cases in Negroes, *Cancer Res* 4:119-127, 1944.
14. Sherman RN, Lee CW, Flynn KJ: Cutaneous squamous cell carcinoma in African-American patients with chronic discoid lupus erythematosus, *Int J Dermatol* 32:677-679, 1993.
15. Weinstock MA: Epidemiology of melanoma, *Cancer Treat Res* 65:29-56, 1993.
16. Katz RD et al: A statistical survey of melanomas of the foot, *JAAD* 28:1008-1011, 1993.

17. Stevens NG, Liff JM, Wess NS: Plantar melanoma: is the incidence of melanoma of the sole really higher in African Amercians than whites? *Int J Cancer* 45:691-693, 1990.

18. Weinstock MA, Horm JW: Mycosis fungoides in the United States, *JAMA* 260:42-46, 1988.

19. Braverman IM: Cutaneous T-cell lymphoma, *Curr Prob Dermatol* 3:184-227, 1991.

20. Gorg SK et al: Dermatofibrosarcoma protuberans: Northern Algeria—a clinicopathologic review of 17 cases, *Clin Oncol* 4:113-122, 1978.

21. Lee B, Mora RG: Kaposi's sarcoma: a comparative analysis in 17 white and 19 African-American patients, *South Med J* 79:540-542, 1985.

22. Phillips JI, Sher R: Kaposi's sarcoma in different populations of South Africa, *S Afr Med J* 71:615-619, 1987.

23. Burkett JM: Dark plaques in nether regions, *JAMA* 230:439-440, 1974.

24. Mora RG, Pernicario C, Lee B: Cancer of the skin in African Americans. III. A review of nineteen African-American patients with Bowen's disease, *J Am Acad Dermatol* 11:557-562, 1984.

Melasma

Gary M. White

Melasma is a common, benign, symmetric facial hyperpigmentation found primarily in women. Its onset is often related to increased sun or hormonal exposure. Standard treatment consists of topical hydroquinone or tretinoin and sun avoidance. Other topical agents, chemical peels, and laser treatments are being evaluated.

ETIOLOGY

The exact cause of melasma is unknown. It is an acquired condition, and is often brought on by pregnancy or the use of oral contraceptives. However, it is a mistake to assume that all or even most patients are so exposed. A woman who is not taking oral contraceptives and who is not pregnant may develop melasma in the setting of significant repeated sun exposure, especially if she is dark skinned. Of note, the use of estrogen in postmenopausal women is not a typical trigger for melasma. Isotretinoin has been reported to induce melasma, but this is undoubtedly rare and resolves in the majority of cases after the retinoid is withdrawn.[1]

A woman who is not taking oral contraceptives and who is not pregnant may develop melasma in the setting of significant repeated sun exposure, especially if she is dark skinned.

Lutfi et al[2] found an association between thyroid autoimmunity and melasma, mostly in women who developed melasma during pregnancy or after use of oral contraceptive drugs. Perez, Sanchez, and Aquilo[3] found evidence of elevated levels of luteinizing hormone in nine patients with melasma and suggested that women with melasma may have subclinical ovarian dysfunction. These results, however, await further corroboration.

EPIDEMIOLOGY

As mentioned, adult females are primarily affected. Men occasionally develop melasma, and their clinical presentation seems to be similar to that of white women.[4] Hormones do not trigger melasma in men. Instead, a genetic predisposition and UV exposure seem to be the most important factors. People of all races may be affected, but those of darker skin color (skin types IV through VI [Box 4-1]) are more susceptible. A positive family history of melasma is typical (with rates reported from 50% to 70%), suggesting a genetic predisposition.

Box 4-1   Fitzpatrick Skin Phototypes

Type I: Always burns easily, shows no immediate pigment darkening, never tans.

Type II: Always burns easily, trace immediate pigment darkening, tans minimally and with difficulty.

Type III: Burns minimally, + immediate pigment darkening, tans gradually and uniformly (light brown).

Type IV: Burns minimally, ++ immediate pigment darkening, tans well (moderate brown).

Type V: Rarely burns, +++ immediate pigment darkening, tans very well (dark brown).

Type VI: Never burns, +++ immediate pigment darkening, tans profusely (black).

From Fitzpatrick TB: *Arch Dermatol* 124:869, 1988.

CLINICAL

Symmetric, uniformly hyperpigmented, sharply defined macules and patches on the face in the sun-exposed areas of a woman are characteristic of melasma (Figures 4-1 and 4-2). It may appear as large patches or confetti-like pigmented macules. Melasma commonly affects the upper lip, cheeks, and forehead. Some women complain of a "mustache" appearance that melasma gives them. Inflammation is absent. Other areas in addition to the face may occasionally be affected, such as the anterior chest, upper back (Figure 4-3), and the photoexposed side of the arms (Figure 4-1). Onset is usually in the summer months when UV exposure is high.

Several clinical presentations have been noted (Table 4-1). The centrofacial variant is characterized by pigmentation primarily of the cheeks, forehead, upper lip, nose, and chin. In the malar variant, pigmented patches are found in the malar regions of the cheeks and nose. Finally, in the mandibular distribution, the pigmented areas are noted along the ramus of the mandible.

A Wood's light examination is valuable in determining the location of the pigment (i.e., epidermal or dermal) because the light accentuates the appearance of the epidermal variant, whereas it does not in the dermal variant. There is also a mixed type of melasma, where both epidermal and dermal pigment are present, and an indeterminate type, so called because the Wood's light cannot be used effectively in such dark (type VI) skin. It should be noted that the location of the pigment may have significant implications with regard to treatment. When the pigmentation is epidermal, it is more "accessible" to treatment and thus shows greater improvement with the various therapies. In the study by Kimbrough-Green et al[5] using tretinoin, the reduction in epidermal pigmentation was statistically greater compared to vehicle, whereas the reduction in dermal pigmentation was not.

When the pigmentation of melasma is epidermal, it is more "accessible" to treatment.

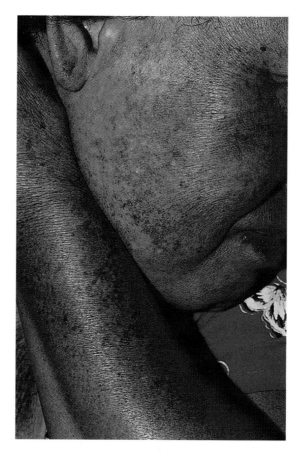

Figure 4-1   Melasma in a Hispanic woman. Note the involvement of the arms as well.

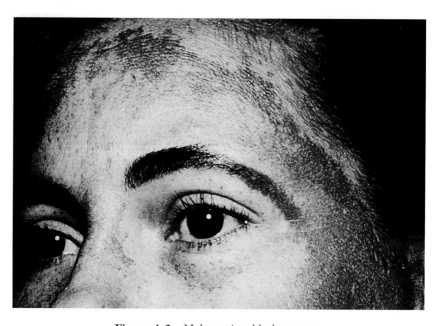

Figure 4-2   Melasma in a black woman.

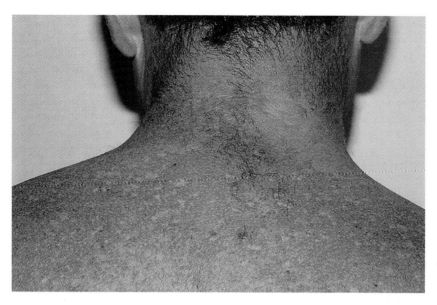

Figure 4-3   Melasma-like pigmentation of the upper back in a man.

Table 4-1   Classification of Melasma

	Predominant patient			
	Puerto Rican men[4]	**Black women[5]**	**White women[8]**	**Hispanic women[6]**
N	27	30	50	76
Average age	39 yrs	53 yrs	42 yrs	39 yrs
Age of onset	31 yrs	41 yrs	30 yrs	29 yrs
Family history	70%	47%	47%	21%
Pattern				
Centrofacial	44%	10%	72%	63%
Malar	44%	73%	14%	21%
Mandibular	11%	17%	14%	16%
Location of Pigment				
Epidermal	67%	43%	94%	72%
Dermal	26%	37%	4%	13%
Mixed or indeterminate	7%	20%	2%	14%

Table 4-1 also compares the characteristics of melasma in different patient populations. Admittedly, these studies are small in size and number, but the trend is that black women are more likely to have the onset of their melasma at an older age and have a malar distribution. The dermal type may also be more common in darker-skinned patients. Also, Kimbrough-Green et al[5] found a small subset of black patients whose melasma was less well marginated than that seen in lighter-skinned patients.

HISTOLOGY

A histologic study of epidermal melasma has revealed prominent melanin deposition in the basal and suprabasal layers. The melanocytes are highly dendritic, anastomosing with each other with arborizing of their dendrites.[4,6] In the dermal type, melanin-laden macrophages are scattered in the superficial dermis without an inflammatory infiltrate.

DIFFERENTIAL DIAGNOSIS

Most cases of melasma are clinically apparent, and a skin biopsy is rarely needed. Postinflammatory hyperpigmentation may be excluded by history. Exogenous ochronosis in the United States is rare indeed, but should always be kept in mind. In some countries, other diseases must be considered. In Nigeria, for example, the differential diagnosis of facial hypermelanosis as recounted by Olumide, Odunowo, and Odiase[7] includes hydroquinone-induced ochronosis, mercury deposition from mercury-containing soaps and creams, systemic drug-induced pigmentation (e.g., clofazimine), photosensitizing herbal concoctions, and facial erythema ab igne in cooks who are exposed to the sun, the heat of an open fire, and various photoactive chemicals for most of the day.

TREATMENT

The need for sun protection should also be discussed. Each patient should be asked, "How much time do you spend in the sun?" It is always helpful to have the patient specify the exact number of minutes during a typical day that she is exposed to the sun. In that way, the 5 minutes walking to and from the car, the 15 minutes outside for lunch, etc., will not be overlooked. Even this minimal exposure is too much for the patient with melasma. Daily morning application of a broad spectrum sunscreen (SPF ≥15) is critical. If the patient is to be out for more than 20 minutes, an SPF 30 or higher sunscreen is recommended. If she is to be out all day, reapplication of a waterproof, SPF 30 or higher sunscreen every 2 hours is recommended. Hats, shade, and other protective measures are also recommended.

Daily morning application of a broad-spectrum sunscreen (SPF ≥15) is critical. If the patient is to be out for more than 20 minutes, an SPF 30 or higher sunscreen is recommended.

Sun protection is usually combined with topical therapy (Box 4-2). Hydroquinone (2% over the counter [OTC] and 3% to 4% prescription) has been used for years as a bleaching agent. It is a phenolic compound that inhibits the conversion of dopa to melanin by inhibiting the tyrosinase enzyme. Hydroquinone has shown positive results for treatment of melasma when given twice daily for 12 weeks. Solaquin Forte, Eldopaque Forte gel or cream, or Melanex solution are all appropriate prescription formulations available in the United States. Solaquin and Eldopaque have sunscreen in them (approximately SPF 18) and therefore are of double value. Alternatively, Melanex may be applied and then covered with a moisturizer that has a sunscreen. Monobenzyl either of hydroquinone, a permanent bleaching agent, should never be used to treat melasma.

Box 4-2   Melasma Therapy

Topical	Surgical
Broad-spectrum sunscreen	Laser*
Hydroquinone (2% over the counter and 3%-4% prescription)	Chemical peel*
Tretinoin	
Azelaic acid	
Alphahydroxy acids*	

*Evolving and/or yet to become standard therapy.

Side effects of hydroquinone are minimal. Local skin irritation may occur, but is uncommon. Hydroquinone has the potential for lightening the surrounding skin. Thus patients should be encouraged to apply the medication only on dark areas. Ochronosis is exceedingly rare in the United States and is discussed elsewhere (see Chapter 17).

Tretinoin 0.1% cream applied at bedtime for 6 to 12 months is also helpful and is effective for melasma in both white[8] and black[5] patients if given over 40 weeks in combination with daily sunscreen use. In practice, however, the 0.1% cream is poorly tolerated by many patients. Indeed, in the study by Griffiths et al,[8] 88% of the tretinoin-treated group (0.1% cream) experienced moderate cutaneous reactions, and in 20% of the patients severe reactions were noted. In addition, there is the risk in dark-skinned patients of inducing a retinoid dermatitis followed by postinflammatory hyperpigmentation. For these reasons, the 0.05% cream or the 0.025% gel is recommended.

Azelaic acid (available in the United States as Azelex; FDA approved for the treatment of acne) is a naturally occurring dicarboxylic acid that is effective in treating melasma when given twice daily for 6 months. It is tolerated very well, and side effects (mainly local skin irritation) are uncommon.

Little is yet known about the benefits of kojic acid, a tyrosinase inhibitor found in the fungus *Aspergillus oryzae*. One study comparing it against hydroquinone (both with glycolic acid) found no measurable difference.[9]

Various combinations using hydroquinone with or without tretinoin and/or a topical steroid have been tried by individual physicians. In 1975 Kligman and Willis[10] reported success in the treatment of melasma with once daily application of a compounded mixture of 5% hydroquinone, 0.1% tretinoin, and 0.1% dexamethasone. They claimed that omission of any one ingredient significantly reduced the clinical effect. This "magic" triple-combination therapy has been variously supported and debunked in the literature. Gano and Garcia[11] reported success with patients applying 0.05% tretinoin cream in the morning, 0.1% betamethasone valerate in the afternoon, and 2% hydroquinone in the evening. Pathak, Fitzpatrick, and Kraus[12] report having tested 300 Hispanic patients using various combinations of hydroquinone, tretinoin, and a topical steroid. They recommend using a compounded cream or lotion containing 2% hydroquinone and 0.05% or 0.1% tretinoin applied twice daily. They found the addition of a steroid unnecessary. Of note, topical clobetasol propionate used as monotherapy in 10 patients cleared much of the pigmentation in 6 to 8 weeks, but side effects prevented long-term use, and recurrence after discontinuation was common.[13] There is always concern about using such a strong steroid on the face for months to years, but on the other hand, tretinoin reduces or prevents the atrophy caused by topical corticosteroid use.

The following general compounding formula may be used, with or without inclusion of a topical steroid. Combine equal parts (e.g., 30 g each) of tretinoin 0.1% cream, hydroquinone 4% cream, and a class VI-III topical steroid cream, if desired. Apply to dark areas of the face twice daily.

Hydroquinone has been recently combined with glycolic acid in commercial formulations, and they are being widely marketed in the United States. The use of this combination has many proponents, yet its true efficacy has yet to be proved in controlled trials.

Summary of Topical Therapy

It has been asserted that hydroquinone is superior to tretinoin in the treatment of melasma because of its lower side effect profile and shorter duration of treatment needed to see significant results (12 weeks for hydroquinone versus 40 weeks for tretinoin).[14] In our view, however, monotherapy is not the usual approach. We recommend using at least two of these medications in combination—usually hydroquinone twice daily with either tretinoin at bedtime or azelaic acid twice daily. Alternatively, a pharmacy-compounded formulation as outlined above may be tried. Every patient must use a broad-spectrum sunscreen every morning and be encouraged to avoid intense periods of UV exposure. Any intervention must be given for 6 to 12 months to determine its full benefit. Patients should be cautioned against expecting quick results. They should also be told to expect 50% lightening over time.

CHEMICAL PEELS AND LASER

Superficial chemical peels have been done successfully in darker-skinned patients, but hyperpigmentation is a significant risk. Hypopigmentation and keloid formation would be risks for medium depth or deep chemical peels (trichloracetic acid or phenol), which are not commonly performed on ethnic skin. Preliminary results of several studies suggest that chemical peels may augment the response to tretinoin and hydroquinone, perhaps by enhancing percutaneous penetration. Excellent clinical results were reported in 16 women with skin types IV, V, and VI who underwent 2 weeks of topical tretinoin 0.05% followed by three superficial peels using either Jessner's solution or a 70% glycolic acid preparation at 1-month intervals.[15] A similar benefit was found when glycolic acid peels were combined with a 2% hydroquinone/10% glycolic acid solution applied daily. It must be emphasized that these preliminary studies require further confirmation.

The Q-switched ruby laser,[16] the 510 nm pigmented lesion dye laser,[17] and the copper vapor laser[18] have all been used to treat melasma with unimpressive or poor results. It remains to be seen if laser treatment will ultimately play a role in the therapy of melasma.

REFERENCES

1. Burke H, Carmichael AJ: Reversible melasma associated with isotretinoin, *Br J Dermatol* 135:862, 1996.
2. Lutfi RJ et al: Association of melasma with thyroid autoimmunity and other thyroidal abnormalities and their relationship to the origin of the melasma, *J Clin Endocrinol Metab* 61:28-31, 1985.
3. Perez M, Sanchez JL, Aquilo F: Endocrinologic profile of patients with idiopathic melasma, *J Invest Dermatol* 81:543-545, 1983.

4. Vázquez M et al: Melasma in men: a clinical and histologic study, *Int J Dermatol* 27:25-27, 1988.
5. Kimbrough-Green CK et al: Topical retinoic acid (tretinoin) for melasma in black patients, *Arch Dermatol* 130:727-733, 1994.
6. Sanchez NP, Pathak MA, Sato S: Melasma: a clinical, light microscopic, ultrastructural, and immunofluorescence study, *J Am Acad Dermatol* 4:698-710, 1981.
7. Olumide YM, Odunowo BD, Odiase AO: Regional dermatoses in the African. Part I. Facial hypermelanosis, *Int J Dermatol* 30:186-189, 1991.
8. Griffiths CE et al: Topical tretinoin (retinoic acid) improves melasma: a vehicle-controlled, clinical trial, *Br J Dermatol* 129:415-421, 1993.
9. Garcia A, Fulton JE: The combination of glycolic acid and hydroquinone or kojic acid for the treatment of melasma and related conditions, *Dermatol Surg* 22:443-447, 1996.
10. Kligman AM, Willis I: A new formula for depigmenting human skin, *Arch Dermatol* 111:40-48, 1975.
11. Gano SE, Garcia RL: Topical tretinoin, hydroquinone and betamethasone valerate in the therapy of melasma, *Cutis* 23:239-241, 1979.
12. Pathak MA, Fitzpatrick TB, Kraus EW: Usefulness of retinoic acid in the treatment of melasma, *J Am Acad Dermatol* 15:894-899, 1986.
13. Kanwar AJ, Dhar S, Kaur S: Treatment of melasma with potent topical steroids, *Dermatol* 188:170, 1994.
14. Grimes PE: Melasma: etiologic and therapeutic considerations, *Arch Dermatol*, 131:1453-1457, 1995.
15. *Skin and Allergy News*, p 20, Feb 1996.
16. Taylor CR, Anderson RR: Ineffective treatment of refractory melasma and postinflammatory hyperpigmentation by Q-switched ruby laser, *J Dermatol Surg Oncol* 20:592-597, 1994.
17. Grekin RC et al: 510-nm pigmented lesion dye laser: its characteristics and clinical uses, *J Dermatol Surg Oncol* 19:380-387, 1993.
18. Goldberg DJ: Benign pigmented lesions of the skin: treatment with the Q-switched ruby laser, *J Dermatol Surg Oncol* 18:376-379, 1993.

Chapter 5

Postinflammatory Pigmentation Disorders

Gary M. White

POSTINFLAMMATORY HYPERPIGMENTATION

Postinflammatory hyperpigmentation is the process whereby dark patches occur at sites of prior inflammation. White persons may be affected by this process, but the changes are much more common and more severe in the darker-skinned patient. Two types of hyperpigmentation occur—epidermal and dermal—based on the location of the pigment. Usually, time and the prevention of the inciting skin condition are the only interventions needed.

Etiology

Two distinct processes seem to cause postinflammatory hyperpigmentation. In the epidermal type, the inciting inflammatory process causes an increase in melanogenesis and the transferring of melanin granules to the surrounding keratinocytes. In the dermal type, disruption and/or destruction of the basal cell layer is followed by phagocytosis of the resultant debris by scavenger macrophages. These pigment-containing macrophages, or *melanophages* as they are called, may persist in the dermis for a time. In some cases, the melanophage seems "stuck" in the dermis, and the pigmentation persists for years.

In the epidermal type, the inciting inflammatory process causes an increase in melanogenesis and the transferring of melanin granules to the surrounding keratinocytes. In the dermal type, disruption and/or destruction of the basal cell layer is followed by phagocytosis of the resultant debris by scavenger macrophages.

How does inflammation stimulate melanogenesis? Tomita, Maeda, and Tagami[1] suggest that various chemical mediators of inflammation (e.g., prostaglandins, thromboxane, leukotriene) may provide the stimulus. Why does inflammation stimulate melanogenesis? Nordlund[2] has hypothesized that the melanocyte plays an integral role in the immune response and thus it is not strange to see pigmentary effects resulting from inflammation. Such theories await further corroboration.

Epidemiology

Many inflammatory diseases in darker-skinned patients can result in hyperpigmentation of the skin. Typical offenders include acne folliculitis, nummular eczema, fixed drug eruptions, the classic maculopapular drug eruption, and lichen planus. Trauma (e.g., scrapes and burns) may also result in the same hyperpigmentation. It is common for the postinflammatory change to be more alarming to the patient or patient's parent than the underlying disorder.

It is common for the postinflammatory change to be more alarming to the patient or patient's parent than the underlying disorder.

Certain diseases tend to cause one pattern preferentially over another. For example, in the controlled study by Bulengo-Ransby et al[3] of postinflammatory hyperpigmentation (the majority of which was caused by acne), pretreatment biopsies showed the melanin to be only epidermal in location. None of the biopsies showed dermal melanin. Surprisingly, there was no significant difference between the dermal melanin content of normal versus postinflammatory hyperpigmentation lesions. In contrast, those processes that disrupt or destroy the basal layer (e.g., lichen planus, lichenoid drug eruption, and fixed drug eruption) often result in the dermal pattern of postinflammatory hyperpigmentation.

The incidence of postinflammatory hyperpigmentation is determined by the incidence of the skin diseases that can cause it and the susceptibility of the patient population, the primary determining factor being the darkness of the skin.

Clinical

A hyperpigmented patch at the exact site of a prior inflammatory condition is typical. The exact shape of the prior lesion is usually formed by the dark spot. Any part of the body, including the face, trunk, and extremities, may be affected. Patients may have one spot or many, depending on the extent of the inciting process. This sort of hyperpigmentation is classically the main manifestation of phytophotodermatitis (Figures 5-1 and 5-2), but may occur after lichen planus, nummular eczema (Figure 5-3), and a variety of other inflammatory dermatoses.

The color of postinflammatory hyperpigmentation of the epidermal type is some shade of brown, whereas that of the dermal type is bluish or slate blue-gray. Use of the Wood's light is particularly helpful in distinguishing epidermal from dermal postinflammatory hyperpigmentation. When viewed with the light, epidermal postinflammatory hyperpigmentation becomes more prominent, whereas dermal postinflammatory hyperpigmentation does not. This attempt to distinguish between the two types is important in that therapy is very much directed by the location of the melanin.

Histology

As mentioned, two patterns of postinflammatory hyperpigmentation may be seen. In the epidermal type, the melanin is epidermal and is often concentrated in the basal layer.[3] In the dermal type, melanin is seen both within and outside dermal melanophages.

Treatment

Preventing further trauma and/or inflammation is critically important in the treatment of postinflammatory hyperpigmentation. Thus the patient with acne desperately needs her acne controlled as much as she needs active treatment of the postinflamma-

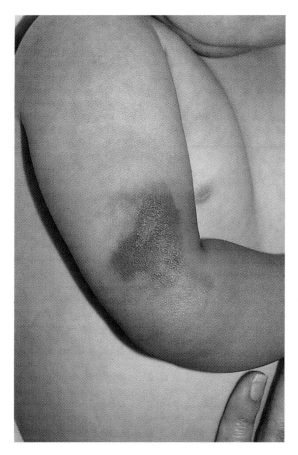

Figure 5-1   Postinflammatory hyperpigmentation in a child several days after going to the beach. The parents were making tropical drinks with lime.

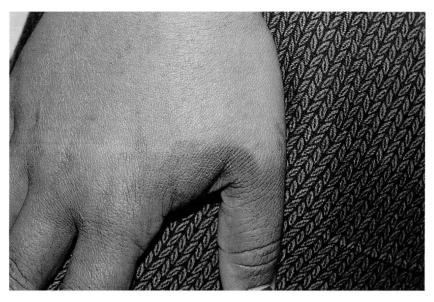

Figure 5-2   Postinflammatory hyperpigmentation in another case of "lime" disease. This pigmented patch occurred several days after going to Mexico and drinking tequila and lime.

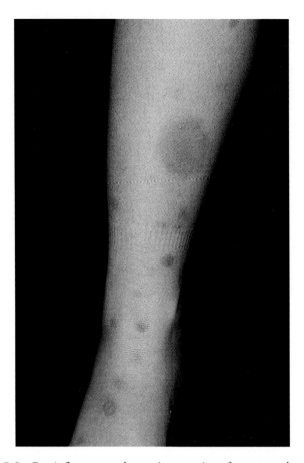

Figure 5-3   Postinflammatory hyperpigmentation after nummular eczema.

tory hyperpigmentation. It is easier to prevent a postinflammatory hyperpigmentation lesion than to remove it once it has formed. If the inciting inflammatory process is controlled, observation is often the only other intervention. Patients should be told that the time it takes for lesions to fade is highly variable. It may be months, years, or possibly never.

Preventing further trauma and/or inflammation is critically important in the treatment of postinflammatory hyperpigmentation. It is easier to prevent a postinflammatory hyperpigmentation lesion than to remove it once it has formed.

If further intervention is desired, and the clinical type is not obvious from the physical examination, a biopsy may be indicated. If the pigment is epidermal in location, there are more potentially helpful treatment options than with dermal postinflammatory hyperpigmentation. Unfortunately, pigment located in the dermis is relatively inaccessible to therapy. Even use of the laser has met with variable and often disappointing results.

Epidermal postinflammatory hyperpigmentation may be treated in a variety of ways. Photoprotection with a broad-spectrum sunscreen (UVA and UVB), protective

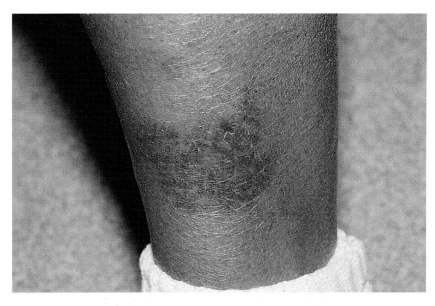

Figure 5-4   Persistent pigmentation in a scar more than a decade old.

clothing, and avoidance of peak UV exposure times are all important. In addition, topical hydroquinone, tretinoin, and azelaic acid may be tried.

Tretinoin (e.g., 0.05% cream) applied at bedtime is effective[4] for epidermal postinflammatory hyperpigmentation and should be combined with sunscreen use if the lesion is on sunexposed skin. Care must be taken not to induce a dermatitis that could contribute to the problem, although Bulengo-Ransby et al[3] found a lower incidence of tretinoin irritation in black subjects than white (50% versus 82%). In that study, they noted a very minimal lightening of normal skin as well.

Azelaic acid (Azelex cream) applied twice daily can cause lightening of hyperpigmented lesions as well. This medication and tretinoin are particularly suited for the acne patient with postinflammatory hyperpigmentation because the drugs are effective against both diseases.[5]

Hydroquinone 2% to 4% is thought to have some benefit in the treatment of epidermal postinflammatory hyperpigmentation, but as with the other medications it must be used diligently for many months, and patients may experience only partial benefit.[6]

It cannot be emphasized enough that prevention of postinflammatory hyperpigmentation is much more beneficial than treating existing lesions. Resolution is often slow, and patients must be counseled accordingly (Figure 5-4).

POSTINFLAMMATORY HYPOPIGMENTATION

Etiology and Pathogenesis

In postinflammatory hypopigmentation, a disease process disturbs the normal pigmentation; as the disease clears, a hypopigmented area is left. The classic example is pityriasis alba, where a patch of eczema causes the pigment lightening, but other diseases (e.g., psoriasis) may do so as well. Some evidence suggests that in pityriasis alba, the keratinocyte is abnormal and unable to accept melanin. For example, Urano–Suehisa, and Tagami[7] studied pityriasis alba using scanning electron microscopy and water-holding capacity analysis. They found that the corneocyte has a smaller surface

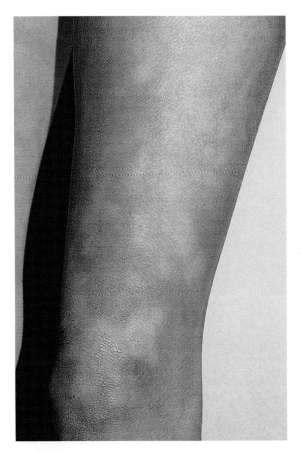

Figure 5-5   Postinflammatory hypopigmentation after a flare of atopic dermatitis.

area and a more prominent villous pattern, suggesting that the skin's water-holding capacity is impaired.

Clinical

A hypopigmented (not depigmented) spot remains in the site of a prior inflammatory process (Figures 5-5 and 5-6). In cases where the initial condition is nearly inapparent, the occurrence of the white spot may be the first thing noted by the patient or parent. This is often true in pityriasis alba.

Treatment

In contrast to postinflammatory hyperpigmentation, the process of postinflammatory hypopigmentation is always epidermal. There is no dermal debris to remove. Thus once the precipitating disease has resolved, normalization of pigmentation should follow in short order (e.g., in 1 to 2 months). It must be emphasized, however, that any presence of the precipitating disease (e.g., xerosis, eczema, psoriasis) should be treated. Any dry skin should be treated with emollient cream once or twice daily. Lotions, with

---

In contrast to postinflammatory hyperpigmentation, the process of postinflammatory hypopigmentation is always epidermal.

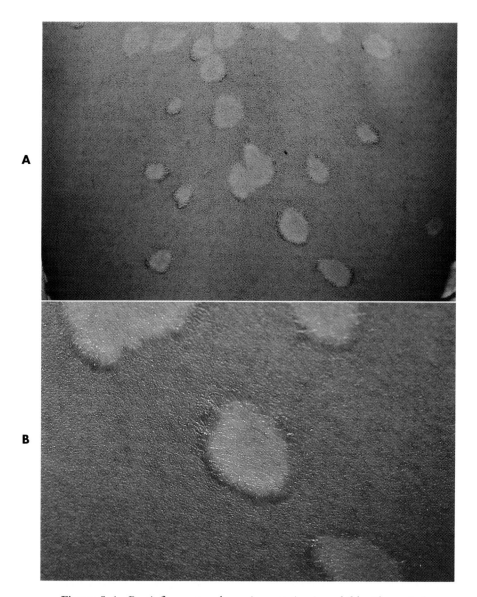

Figure 5-6   Postinflammatory hypopigmentation in a child with psoriasis.

their high water content, are less effective. If any erythema suggesting persistent inflammation is present, a topical steroid should be prescribed. For young children with pityriasis alba of the face, hydrocortisone 1% cream is effective (see Pityriasis Alba, p 149).

REFERENCES

1. Tomita Y, Maeda K, Tagami H: Mechanisms for hyperpigmentation in postinflammatory pigmentation, urticaria pigmentosa and sunburn, *Dermatologica* (Suppl 1) 179:49-53, 1989.
2. Nordlund JJ: Postinflammatory hyperpigmentation, *Dermatol Clin* 6:185-192, 1988.
3. Bulengo-Ransby SM et al: Topical tretinoin (retinoic acid) therapy for hyperpigmented lesions caused by inflammation of the skin in black patients, *N Engl J Med* 328:1438-1443, 1993.

4. LaVoo EJ: Tretinoin for hyperpigmentation in black patients, *N Engl J Med* 329:1503, 1993.
5. Epstein JH: Postinflammatory hyperpigmentation, *Clin Dermatol* 7:55-65, 1989.
6. Engasser PG, Maibach HI: Cosmetic and dermatology: bleaching creams, *J Am Acad Dermatol* 5:143, 1981.
7. Urano-Suehisa S, Tagami H: Functional and morphological analysis of the horny layer of pityriasis alba, *Acta Derm Venereol* 65:164-167, 1985.

Normal Skin Changes in the Black Patient

Gary M. White

HYPERPIGMENTED MACULES OF THE PALMAR CREASES

Pigmented macules are commonly seen on the palms and soles of black patients (Figure 6-1). Darker-skinned blacks seem to be more frequently affected than those with lighter skin. Very few studies have been done, but in one, 87 of 145 (60%) adult black patients were found to have volar pigmented macules.[1] They varied in size from 2 mm to several centimeters in diameter. Histologic examination showed epidermal pigmentation of all layers, with the melanin residing in large dendritic melanocytes. No treatment is needed. The etiology is unknown.

LEUKOEDEMA

Leukoedema is a common, benign condition of the oral mucosa of black adults. Archard and Stanley[2] concluded from a histologic analysis that the clinical changes are a result of a retained layer of parakeratotic cells.

Etiology

The cause of leukoedema is unknown, although some have hypothesized that irritation and/or poor oral hygiene are causative or triggering factors. Several studies have looked at the correlation with smoking, and both negative[3] and positive[4] results have been found. Axéll, Andersson, and Lårsson[5] found that all 18 patients studied who used chewing tobacco and held it against the buccal mucosa had discrete changes of leukoedema there. Other activities reported to induce leukoedema include cannabis smoking, cheek sucking, betel nut chewing, and coca leaf chewing.[6]

Epidemiology

Most reports emphasize the higher incidence of leukoedema in darker-skinned patients, but this may be a result of the ease with which leukoedema is observed on a pigmented background. The true incidence of this condition remains in question, but it probably depends on how hard one looks. Using an intense examination light, Durocher, Thalman, and Fiore-Donno[7] found some changes of leukoedema in 97% of their population (almost all of whom were white). Some studies have shown a slight male preference.

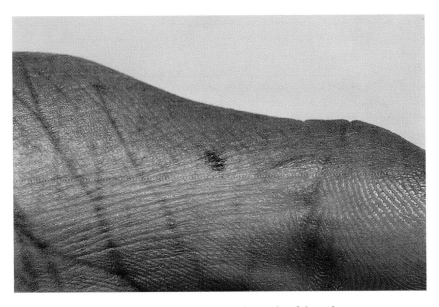

Figure 6-1   Hyperpigmented macule of the palm.

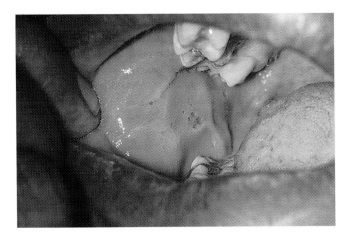

Figure 6-2   Leukoedema.

Most reports emphasize the higher incidence of leukoedema in darker-skinned patients, but this may be a result of the ease with which leukoedema is observed on a pigmented background.

Clinical

Clinical examination of the oral mucosa affected by leukoedema shows it to have a white-grey, edematous surface that has been described as "filmy opalescence" (Figure 6-2). The buccal mucosa is primarily involved, especially the middle and posterior areas, but the lingual mucosa may be involved as well. This change may cover the majority of the mucosa or may occur in large, ill-defined patches. In well-formed lesions, impressions of the teeth are prominently seen along the occlusal line. The surface is soft, but scraping does not remove the changes. The condition is asymptomatic except for the rare patient who complains of the involved mucosa being caught during mastication.[8] Similar changes have been reported on the mucosa of the lip, uvula, tongue, and vagina.

Clinical examination of the oral mucosa affected by leukoedema shows it to have a white-grey, edematous surface that has been described as "filmy opalescence."

Histology

Some controversy exists with regard to the central pathologic features of leukoedema. Intracellular edema (Figure 6-3) is frequently mentioned and is diagnostic for some, but Archard and Stanley[2] argue that this change is normal for mucosal epithelium. They instead rely on the presence of a retained superficial layer of parakeratotic cells. They note that the epithelium is thickened, and this is in large part caused by this retained parakeratotic layer.

Differential Diagnosis

The diagnosis is usually apparent, and a biopsy is rarely needed. The differential diagnosis of white lesions on the oral mucosa includes leukoplakia, white sponge nevus, *Candida*, and lichen planus. Leukoplakia, a potentially premalignant condition, presents as a fixed, white, hyperkeratotic lesion. It is usually not as edematous or opalescent as leukoedema. White sponge nevus is a rare, fixed lesion composed of thick, spongelike plaques. The whitish material of *Candida* can be removed with a tongue blade, whereas leukoedema cannot. Lichen planus of the oral mucosa is distinctly reticular and does not have the pearly, opalescent appearance of leukoedema.

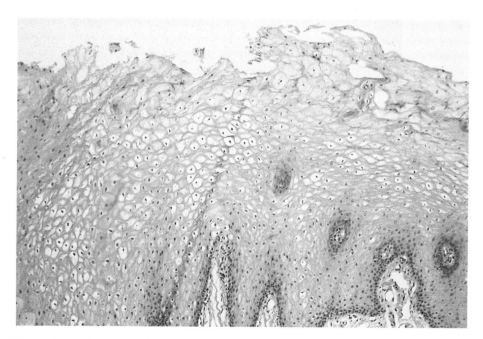

Figure 6-3 Histology of leukoedema. Edematous acanthotic mucosal epithelium, showing parakeratotic cells on the surface. (×400.) (Courtesy Jeffrey C.B. Stewart, DDS, MS, Assistant Professor of Pathology, University of Pennsylvania, School of Dental Medicine.)

Treatment

No treatment is necessary, although cessation of smoking and improvement of oral hygiene may be recommended if appropriate. Topical tretinoin brought about pronounced improvement over 2 weeks in one patient.[8] The condition is not premalignant.

LONGITUDINAL MELANONYCHIA

Longitudinal pigmented stripes of the nails, called *longitudinal melanonychia*, are common in black patients (Figure 6-4). They represent increased production of melanin by melanocytes in the nail matrix. Their numbers often increase, and their appearance darkens with advancing age. Darker-skinned blacks seem to be more commonly affected.

Clinical

Clinical examination shows a pigmented stripe running longitudinally along the nail. The density of pigment is uniform longitudinally, but may vary transversely. The width varies and may increase over time. The thumb and index finger are favored digits.

The primary task of the clinician is to exclude malignancy because an atypical nevus or, rarely, a melanoma of the matrix may cause a longitudinal band. Those lesions that are solitary, wider than 6 mm, dark, and/or have significant variation in pigment

---

The primary task of the clinician is to exclude malignancy because an atypical nevus or, rarely, a melanoma of the matrix may cause a longitudinal band.

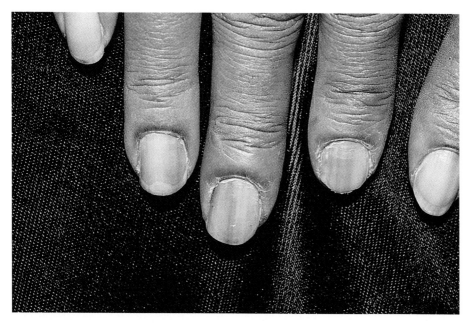

Figure 6-4 Longitudinal melanonychia. These multiple, lightly pigmented bands are not of clinical concern.

are particularly worrisome and should be biopsied. Dystrophy or destruction of any portion of the nail demands a biopsy. Pigmentation of the periungual skin (Hutchinson's sign) is particularly worrisome. A biopsy is performed as follows: make longitudinal incisions of the proximal nail fold on either side of the streak, retract the proximal nail fold, and biopsy the origin of the streak.

Treatment

Treatment is not needed nor is it available.

PIGMENTARY DEMARCATION LINES

Pigmentary demarcation lines (PDLs) most commonly occur in black patients, but have also been described in Asians and even in white patients (Table 6-1). Some authors have expanded the classification of PDLs to include those without a sharp transition from light to dark. This section limits itself to those with a sharp transition, the so-called *types A and B PDLs*. Both *Voigt's lines* and *Futcher's lines* are terms that have been used to describe these changes. One theory suggests that the purpose of PDLs is protection. The dorsal skin is more heavily pigmented to provide the skin better protection from the sun.

One theory suggests that the purpose of PDLs is protection. The dorsal skin is more heavily pigmented to provide the skin better protection from the sun.

Epidemiology

The reported prevalence of these changes varies greatly depending on the source and the population studied. Many black neonates have one or both lines, and the prevalence increases with age. In the study by James, Carter, and Rodman,[9] about 50% of black women and about 33% of black men had type A PDLs. Similarly, about 50% of black women and about 33% of black men had type B PDLs. In the Japanese population, the incidence of type A PDLs was reported to be 39% in females and 23% in males in a study of 1338 subjects by Maruyama.[10] In contrast, a study by Ito[11] of 3000 Japanese reported the overall incidence of type A PDLs to be 6.3%, with many more women affected than men.

Clinical

Type A PDLs are characterized by an abrupt transition between lighter and darker skin on the anterior portion of the upper arms (Figure 6-5). Type B lines are similar in appearance, but occur on the posterior legs. In both, the darker skin is lateral and the lighter skin is medial.

Rarely, a dorsal counterpart of type A PDLs may be seen on the posterior aspect of the upper outer arm. Of note, type B lines may appear or darken with pregnancy[12] and have been reported in black, Hispanic, and white women. At times, an erythema is associated with development of the pigmentation in pregnancy.[13] Some patients experience complete resolution between the first and third months postpartum.

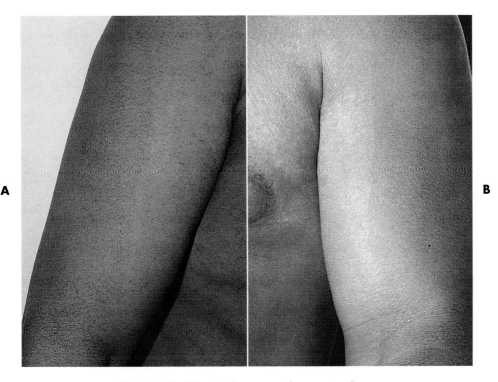

Figure 6-5   Type A pigmentary demarcation lines.

Table 6-1   An Expanded Classification of Pigmentary Alterations

Type	Description
A	Abrupt transition from darker lateral skin to lighter medial skin on the upper anterior arms
B	Abrupt transition from darker lateral skin to lighter medial skin on the posterior legs
C	Vertical hypopigmented line in the presternal and parasternal areas
D	Posteromedial area of spine
E	Well-defined hypopigmented patches, most often running from the middle third of the clavicle to periareolar skin

Treatment

PDLs have no clinical significance other than cosmetic considerations. No treatment is available, but thankfully treatment is not needed.

OTHER PIGMENTARY CHANGES

The concept of PDLs has been expanded by some authors beyond the classic types A and B to include hypopigmented areas where an abrupt transition is not seen. Table 6-1 outlines an extended classification of pigmentary alterations.

Midline hypopigmentation (type C) is quite common, occurring in approximately one third of black adults.[9] White patients may also rarely be affected. Well-defined hypopigmented patches running from the middle third of the clavicle to periareolar skin (type E) occur in approximately 13% to 16% of adult black patients. Posterior medial changes in pigmentation (type D) are the least common of these pigmentary alterations, occurring in less than 10% of black adults.

PIGMENTED GUMS

Pigmentation of the oral mucosa is common in the darker-skinned races (Figure 6-6). Various studies have determined the incidence to be approximately 75% to 100% of black patients, and the pigmentation appears in both infants and adults. It is most commonly seen on the gingivae, but may also occur on the hard palate, buccal mucosa, and tongue (Figure 6-7).

Intraoral pigmentation is most commonly seen on the gingivae, but may also occur on the hard palate, buccal mucosa, and tongue.

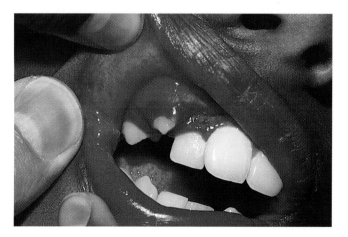

Figure 6-6 Racial pigmentation of the gums.

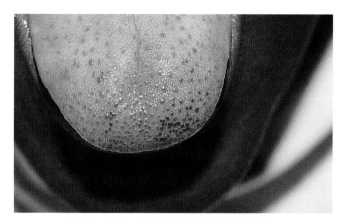

Figure 6-7 Pigmented fungiform papillae of the tongue. Black, pigmented papilla of the tongue, most common in black patients, may occur.

A band-shaped, brownish pigmentation that runs horizontally just above the gingiva is common in Asian children. Mishiro et al[14] found it in 46% of Chinese children and 28% of Japanese children.

No treatment is needed, but periodontists have reported success with a process similar to dermabrasion.[15]

PUNCTATE KERATOSIS OF PALMAR CREASES

Black patients may develop small, hyperkeratotic plugs or, if the plugs are removed, shallow pits in the large creases of the palms and fingers (Figure 6-8). The soles may also be involved. Manual labor and atopy have been reported as associations, but this remains to be confirmed. Both sporadic and familial cases occur. No treatment is needed nor is one known to be effective.[16]

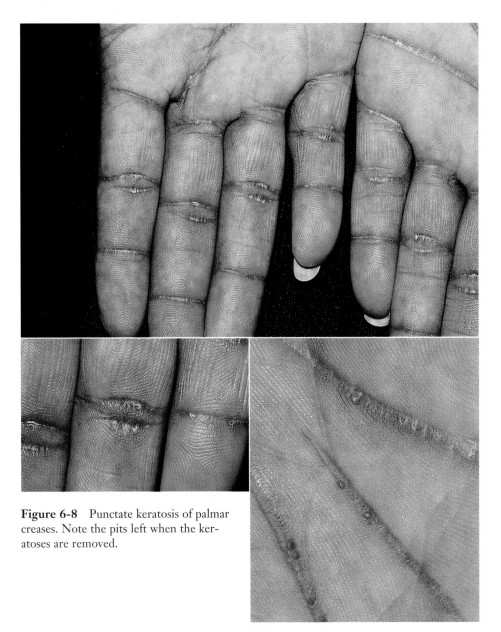

Figure 6-8 Punctate keratosis of palmar creases. Note the pits left when the keratoses are removed.

REFERENCES

1. Chapel TA, Taylor RM, Pinkus H: Volar melanotic macules, *Int J Dermatol* 18:222-225, 1979.
2. Archard HO, Stanley HR: Leukoedema of the oral mucosa: comments on article, *J Am Dent Assoc* 86:300-301, 1973.
3. van Wyk CW: An investigation into the association between leukoedema and smoking, *J Oral Pathol* 14:491-499, 1985.
4. Zain RB, Razak IA: Association between cigarette smoking and prevalence of oral mucosal lesions among Malaysian army personnel, *Community Dent Oral Epidemiol* 17:148-149, 1989.
5. Axéll T, Andersson G, Lårsson A: Oral mucosal findings associated with chewing tobacco in Sweden: a clinical and histological study, *J Dent Assoc South Afr* 47:194, 1992.
6. Darling MR, Arendorf TM: Effects of cannabis smoking on oral soft tissues, *Community Dent Oral Epidemiol* 21:78-81, 1993.
7. Durocher RT, Thalman R, Fiore-Donno G: Leukoedema of the oral mucosa, *J Am Dent Assoc* 85:1105-1109, 1972.
8. Duncan SC, Su D: Leukoedema of the oral mucosa, *Arch Derm* 116:906-908, 1980.
9. James WD, Carter JM, Rodman OG: Pigmentary demarcation lines: a population survey, *J Am Acad Dermatol* 16:584-590, 1987.
10. Maruyama as cited by Miura O: The demarcation lines of pigmentation observed among the Japanese on the inner sides of their extremities and on anterior and posterior sides of their medial regions, *Tohoku J Exp Med* 54:135-140, 1951.
11. Ito K: The peculiar demarcation of pigmentation along the so-called Voight's line among the Japanese, *Dermatol Int* 4:45-47, 1965.
12. James WD et al: Pigmentary demarcation lines associated with pregnancy, *J Am Acad Dermatol* 11:438-440, 1984.
13. Hashimoto K et al: Pigmentary demarcation lines associated with pregnancy in Japanese, *J Dermatol* 12:283-285, 1985.
14. Mishiro Y et al: Gingival pigmentation in preschool children of Chengdu, West China, *J Pedodont* 14:150-151, 1990.
15. Farnoosh AA: Treatment of gingival pigmentation and discoloration for esthetic purposes, *Int J Periodont Restor Dent* 10:312-319, 1990.
16. Weiss RM, Rasmussen JE: Keratosis punctata of the palmar creases, *Arch Dermatol* 116:669-671, 1980.

Diseases

Common Diseases in the Darker-Skinned Adult

Gary M. White

Making a dermatologic diagnosis is often more difficult with a dark-skinned patient because subtle changes in skin color may be hidden. Pink and light red hues may be totally missed. Dark reds and browns may appear as purple, grey, or black. Even more difficult is trying to make an accurate diagnosis after the acute episode when only hypopigmentation or hyperpigmentation remains. Guesses may be made, but often the patient must be told to call if the lesions reappear. Patient history, distribution of lesions, and skin surface changes become more important diagnostic tools.

ACANTHOMA FISSURATUM

Acanthoma fissuratum appears as a papulonodule or plaque in the retroauricular fold, often with a groove where the frames of eyeglasses rest (Figure 7-1). In a white person this lesion may mimic a basal cell carcinoma, but in a black patient such confusion does not occur.

ACNE

Acne vulgaris, or common acne, occurs in blacks as well as whites, but there may be some variation in incidence and manifestations. Wilkins and Voorhees[1] have found a significantly lower incidence of inflammatory acne in blacks than in whites. They studied male prisoners ages 15 to 21. Five percent of 893 white inmates, compared with 0.5% of 753 black inmates, had nodulocystic (grades 3 and 4) acne. Kaidbey and Kligman[2] found that young black males were more likely than whites to form comedones in response to occlusion of 25% crude coal tar on the back. They conclude that in blacks, the follicle is more likely to respond by hyperkeratosis than by disintegration, which is more typical for whites. They also postulate that the black follicle is more "sturdy," and thus much less likely to develop a large, inflammatory nodule because follicular rupture is required for this process. To support this theory, they also point out that pomade acne, which is characteristic of black skin, is primarily a noninflammatory comedonal disease. In this model of acne induced by crude coal tar, the bacteria *Propionibacterium acnes* was absent. Thus one might speculate that in white patients the rupture of the follicle causing the inflammatory nodule may occur from a combination of *P. acnes*-induced host immune attack plus a not very sturdy follicle. In contrast, for black patients, more inflammation and stress must be put on the follicle to cause rupture.

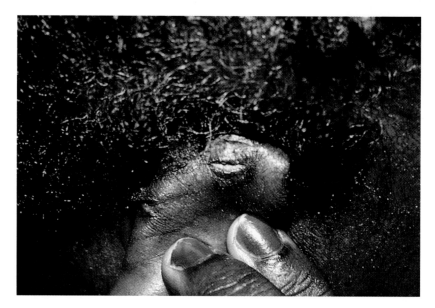

Figure 7-1 Acanthoma fissuratum. This dark plaque has a groove where the frames of the eyeglasses sit. (Courtesy Michael O. Murphy, MD.)

Some new evidence has come to light recently. Halder et al[3] have recently challenged the notion that inflammation is much more common in white patients than in black patients. They photographed and then biopsied facial acne lesions on approximately 30 adult black women. They found that there was a marked inflammation *histologically* in all types of lesions. Their study strongly suggests that inflammation is actually quite common in darker-skinned patients. It only seems uncommon because it is well-hidden.

The other finding from this study that deserves mention concerns the postinflammatory hyperpigmented macules that are so bothersome to darker-skinned patients with acne. Halder et al[3] found that much of the melanin, if not the majority, is epidermal. This finding stands in contrast to the old notion that postinflammatory hyperpigmentation is merely dermal melanin. An earlier study by Bulengo-Ransby et al[4] of postinflammatory hyperpigmented macules, the majority of which were caused by acne, supports this finding. In that study, pretreatment biopsies showed the melanin to be only epidermal in location. None of the biopsies showed dermal melanin in amounts higher than normal skin. The important conclusion here is that such a superficial localization makes these dark spots more accessible to topical therapy. Thus azelaic acid and tretinoin might be particularly helpful here because they both improve acne and decrease hyperpigmentation. Hydroquinone may be helpful as well.

A study by Pochi and Strauss[5] of the sebaceous gland activity of blacks compared with whites did not show any difference.

Clinical

Children from ages 10 to 13 will initially develop comedonal acne (blackheads and whiteheads) of the central face as pubertal hormones surge (Figures 7-2 and 7-3). The facial skin becomes more oily at the same time. This rise in comedonal acne seems to be caused by the hormonal rise in DHEA-S and is an early sign of puberty. Later, inflammatory lesions may occur (Figure 7-4). These lesions are characterized by papules and pustules that on resolution often leave pigmented macules (Figure 7-5). Pitted

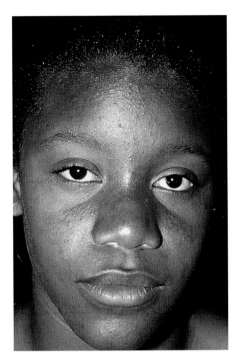

Figure 7-2   Mild acne.

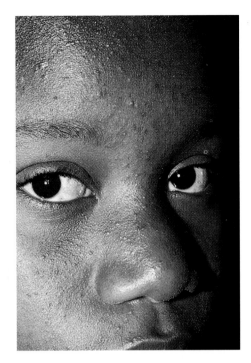

Figure 7-3   Acne. Note the oily skin.

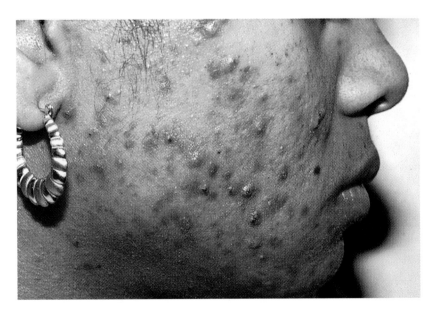

Figure 7-4   Moderate inflammatory acne. This patient was on oral antibiotics and topical therapy at the time of the photograph. She went on to receive a course of isotretinoin.

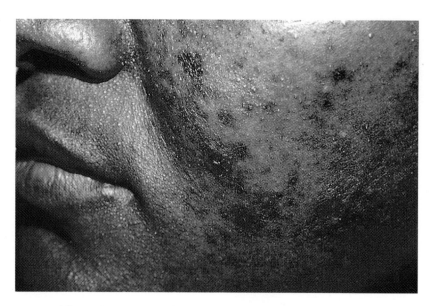

Figure 7-5   Acne with postinflammatory hyperpigmentation.

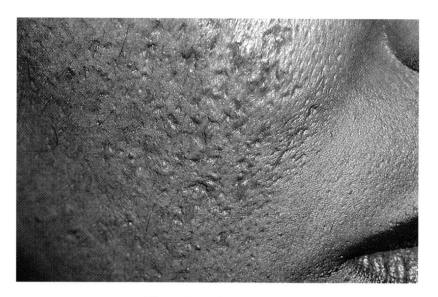

Figure 7-6   Acne scarring.

scars (Figure 7-6) and even keloid scarring (Figure 7-7) may occur. There is an uncommon variant called *infantile acne* that may occur in young children, particularly boys (Figure 7-8). Several specific clinical patterns are common in black patients.

Pomade Acne

The classic patient with pomade acne is black, with innumerable comedones along the hairline and temples. Because of their unique hair type, black patients tend to shampoo less frequently than white patients and apply more oils, greases, and waxes. Some

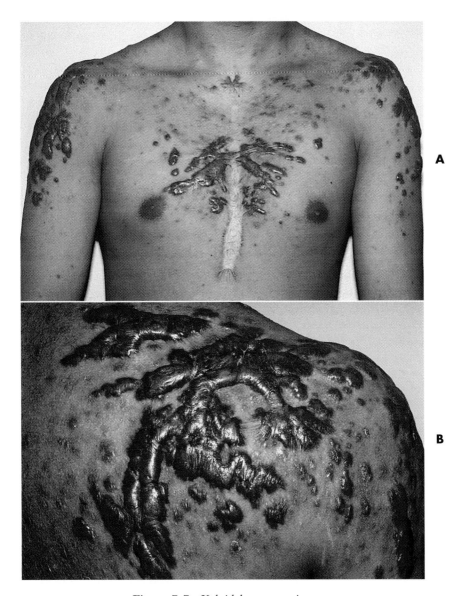

Figure 7-7   Keloidal acne scarring.

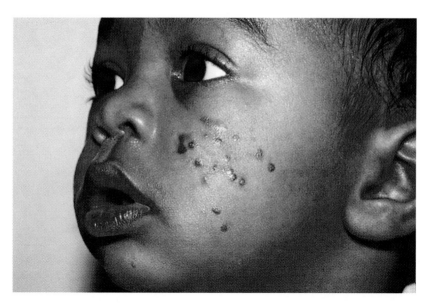

Figure 7-8   Infantile acne. Rarely, the typical inflammatory papules, pustules, and even nodules may present in a child, usually a male, at 3 to 6 months of age. Congenital adrenal hyperplasia or a virilizing tumor should be excluded.

of these are comedogenic and thus induce the characteristic follicular response. Verhagen[6] reports that even young black children between 1 and 12 years old may develop pomade acne. He notes that treating "vaselinoderma" was a signficant part of his practice in Kenya. This condition was caused by the widespread practice of applying petroleum jelly to the faces of African children. It should be remembered that all races can be affected by pomade acne. In the United States, for example, many white teenagers are affected by "pomade acne" because the use of both after-shampoo conditioners and shampoo-conditioner combination products is quite prevalent.

Patient education is required. However, the doctor must take care to show due consideration for the patient's special hair needs and not make unreasonable treatment recommendations such as, "you can't use any oily products in your hair." To minimize the production of acne lesions, nongreasy pomades, such as those with glycerins or silicon oils, are recommended. The patient may also be advised to apply the hair grease every other day. Applying tretinoin, adapalene, or another retinoid every other night, and progressing to nightly use if tolerated, is helpful. Washing the face twice a day with a salicylic acid–containing acne cleanser may be advised as well.

Postinflammatory Hyperpigmentation

Black patients with acne usually complain first of their "scars" or dark spots where the acne once was. These spots are not scars but actually postinflammatory hyperpigmentation. A brown macule at the site of a prior acne lesion in a dark-skinned patient is characteristic. Often patients complain more of this lesion than of the acne. Patients will often use an OTC hydroquinone (e.g., Esoterica) as treatment.

Controlling acne is imperative to preventing new lesions. Using a topical retinoid (e.g., Retin-A, Differin, Avita) and sunscreen and avoiding the sun causes significant

---

Black patients with acne usually complain first of their "scars" or dark spots where the acne once was. These spots are not scars but actually postinflammatory hyperpigmentation.

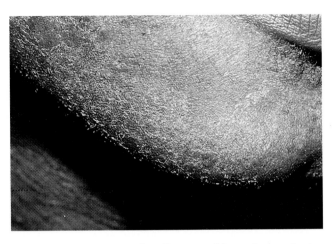

Figure 7-9 Dryness and peeling caused by topical tretinoin.

Table 7-1 Acne Treatments

Acne condition	Therapy
Mild comedonal acne	Salicylic acid cleanser Topical retinoid at bedtime (e.g., Differin, Retin-A Micro, Avita) Topical antimicrobial in the morning (e.g., benzoyl peroxide, clindamycin, benzamycin)
Pomade acne	All of the above, plus reduce or eliminate greasy products from the hair
Moderate acne	All of the above, plus an oral antibiotic such as tetracycline 500 mg twice daily, doxycycline 100 mg twice daily, or minocycline 50-100 mg twice daily
Postinflammatory hyperpigmentation	All of the above, plus daily morning sunscreen (e.g., SPF 15); make sure the acne regimen includes one of the following: azelaic acid twice daily, tretinoin at bedtime
Severe acne	If conventional therapy that includes at least two 6-week courses of two different oral antibiotics plus topical therapy fails, consider Accutane; Accutane should be given at approximately 1 mg/kg for 18 to 20 weeks

lightening of these lesions over time but may also cause dryness and peeling of the skin (Figure 7-9).[7] Azelaic acid may also be beneficial, and is helpful both for acne and hyperpigmentation.

Treatment

Mild comedonal acne is best treated with a topical retinoid to be applied at bedtime and an antimicrobial agent (e.g., clindamycin, benzoyl peroxide) for use in the morning (Table 7-1). Many black patients with acne are concerned that some of the topical medications will alter the color of their skin. Benzoyl peroxide may bleach the carpet and sheets, but there is no evidence that benzoyl peroxide alters the color of the skin (other than through the mechanism of irritation). If significant irritation develops with the use of Retin-A, significant hyperpigmentation can result. Thus less irritating formulations of tretinoin (e.g., Avita) or adapalene are recommended. If irritation does not occur, tretinoin seems to "normalize" skin tone in a sense, making darker skin

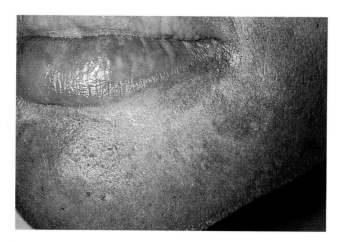

Figure 7-10 An "ashy" appearance caused by oral isotretinoin.

lighter and lighter skin darker. Finally, azelaic acid, although able to lighten hyperpigmentation is thought to rarely lighten normally dark skin.

Acne Vulgaris: Moderate, Papulopustular

For moderate to severe acne, oral antibiotics should be given in conjunction with topical medication (Table 7-1). The options include tetracycline 500 mg twice daily, doxycycline 50 to 100 mg twice daily, and minocycline 50 to 100 mg twice daily. Less commonly used alternatives include erythromycin 500 mg twice daily or 333 mg three times a day, trimethoprim-sulfamethoxazole double-strength formulations (e.g., Septra DS) initially twice daily then tapered to once daily, and amoxicillin 500 mg twice daily. The choice is often based on cost, what has been tried before, and if the patient wants to take the medication on a full or empty stomach. The alleged decrease in effectiveness of oral contraceptives by the above oral antibiotics has not yet been proved but is a theoretical possibility and should be discussed with the patient.

Acne Vulgaris: Severe or Treatment-Resistant

Black patients seem to find themselves in need of Accutane much less often than white patients. This probably relates to factors discussed early in the chapter. Nevertheless, if a patient's acne is not well controlled after a trial of at least two 6-week courses of two different oral antibiotics used in conjunction with topical therapy, Accutane should be considered. It is usually given over an 18- to 20-week course at a dose of 1 mg/kg/day. To save money, a 135-lb woman (approximately 60 kg) may receive 40 mg on even days and 80 mg (two 40-mg capsules) on odd days. All appropriate guidelines should be followed, including educating all patients about common side effects such as dry, chapped lips; dry face (Figure 7-10); muscle aches; backache; dry skin patches on the arms; and headaches.

Black patients seem to find themselves in need of Accutane much less often than white patients. Nevertheless, if a patient's acne is not well controlled after a trial of at least two 6-week courses of two different oral antibiotics used in conjunction with topical therapy, Accutane should be considered.

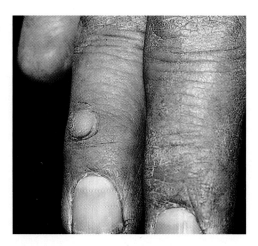

Figure 7-11   Acquired digital fibrokeratoma.

Patients should be warned to watch for serious but uncommon side effects, such as decreased night vision, the worst headache they have ever had, and abdominal pain. Female patients should be referred to a gynecologist for contraceptive counseling. Physicians should be sure that female patients use at least two reliable forms of birth control or are abstinent, get a baseline pregnancy test, and repeat the pregnancy test monthly.

ACQUIRED DIGITAL FIBROKERATOMA

A flesh-colored papule on the finger—usually the index or middle finger—with an epidermal collarette at the base is characteristic of acquired digital fibrokeratoma (Figure 7-11). Occasionally the papules may be warty or pedunculated. These lesions may also occur on the toes, palms, or the heel. No treatment is needed, but simple shave excision is effective for removal.

ALLERGIC CONTACT DERMATITIS

It appears that black patients are affected by allergic contact dermatitis (Figures 7-12 to 7-14) just as are other races, although the frequency of allergic responses may differ. Typical allergens include nickel, paraphenylenediamine, chromates, and mercaptobenzothiazole. Patch testing is performed just as it is with white skin.

It appears that black patients are affected by allergic contact dermatitis just as are other races, although the frequency of allergic responses may differ.

The answer to the question, "is irritant contact dermatitis less common in black versus white skin?" is much more controversial. Several studies have concluded that black skin is less subject to irritation, but as Fischer[8] points out, these results are questionable because erythema, their primary measurement of irritancy, is more difficult to detect in black skin.

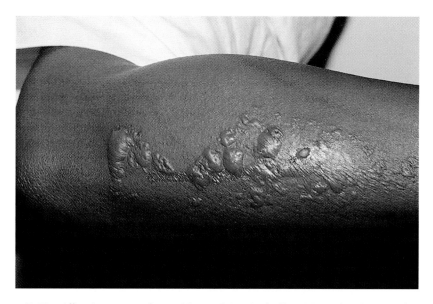

Figure 7-12   Allergic contact dermatitis resulting in bullae. Note the sharp and angular margination.

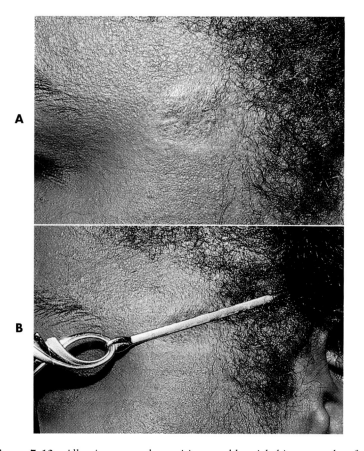

Figure 7-13   Allergic contact dermatitis caused by nickel in an eyeglass frame.

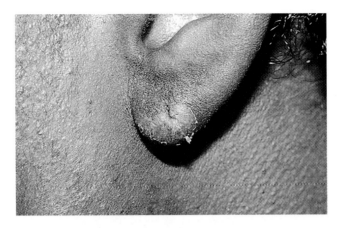

Figure 7-14   Allergic contact dermatitis caused by nickel in earrings.

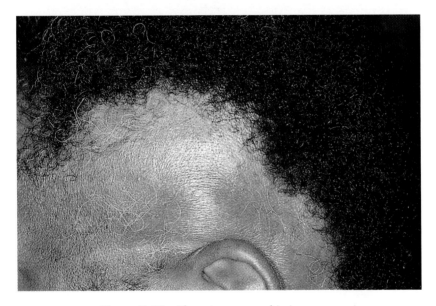

Figure 7-15   Alopecia areata, ophiasis pattern.

ALOPECIA AREATA

Alopecia areata is a nonscarring alopecia that usually presents as round circles of hair loss. More diffuse alopecia or an ophiasis pattern (Figure 7-15) may also occur. (See Chapter 20 for more discussion.)

BACTERIAL FOLLICULITIS

Clinical

Pyodermas (e.g., staphylococcal folliculitis) are quite common in black patients. A bacterial folliculitis presents as multiple follicular pustules. In the dark-skinned patient, the typical erythema may be masked. Hyperpigmented papules (Figure 7-16) and/or pustules with only slight erythema may be the only clinical sign.

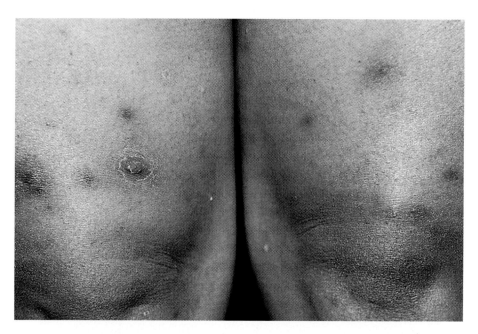

Figure 7-16   Bacterial folliculitis. Hyperpigmented papules with slight erythema are seen.

Figure 7-17   Capillary hemangioma.

CAPILLARY HEMANGIOMAS

Typical red, capillary hemangiomas may occasionally be seen on a black person's skin (Figure 7-17).

CONFLUENT AND RETICULATED PAPILLOMATOSIS

Clinical

Confluent and reticulated brown papules occurring in the midchest area are characteristic of papillomatosis, an uncommon disease (Figure 7-18). These papules may also involve the back, neck, abdomen, axilla, and inframammary area.

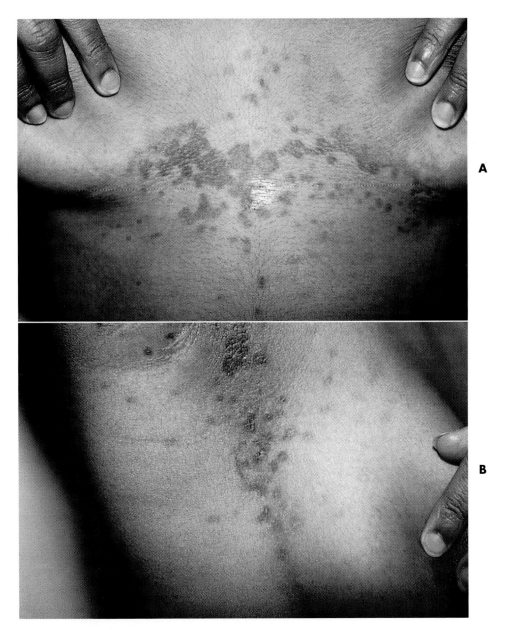

Figure 7-18 Confluent and reticulated papillomatosis. The midline area of the chest is a common location for these confluent and reticulated papules. (Courtesy Michael O. Murphy, MD.)

Treatment

No treatment is needed for this benign disease, although most patients desire treatment for cosmetic reasons. Minocycline 100 mg twice daily for 1 to 3 months[9] has been very effective in many cases and indeed should be considered first-line therapy. The response to retinoids may be dramatic, but temporary, with the disease returning when therapy is discontinued. Topical tretinoin may be effective locally, but for widespread clearing isotretinoin or etretinate may be used.

CONNECTIVE TISSUE DISEASES

Discoid Lupus Erythematosus

Discoid lupus erythematosus (DLE) is the primarily cutaneous form of lupus erythematosus (LE) and is characterized by inflammatory and potentially scarring lesions of sun-exposed areas. Blacks are commonly affected by both DLE and systemic lupus erythematosis (SLE). The pigmentary changes that occur can be very cosmetically disfiguring.

Clinical

The black patient with DLE usually presents with scaly, hyperkeratotic, inflammatory lesions on the sun-exposed areas of the face (Figure 7-19) and arms (Figures 7-20 to 7-22). The correct diagnosis is often missed. Seborrheic dermatitis or eczema are commonly presumed diagnoses. Inflammation, scarring, and alopecia are also typical (Figure 7-23). The inner part of the pinna is commonly affected as well. The scale may fill the follicular orifices and, if confluent, may be peeled back and the undersurface found to resemble the undersurface of a carpet tack (the so-called *carpet-tack sign*). Lesions present for months to years often develop central white scarring with a hyperpigmented border. Squamous cell carcinoma may develop in a longstanding DLE scar.

Children are rarely affected by DLE. According to George and Tunnessen,[10] the presentation and course in children are similar to adult DLE, but there is a lack of female predominance, a low incidence of photosensitivity, and frequent progression to systemic lupus erythematosus (SLE).

Workup

SLE should be excluded by the absence of the American College of Rheumatology criteria for diagnosis of SLE. Workup should include a history and physical, CBC,

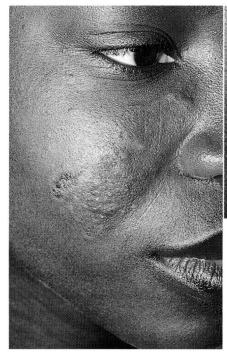
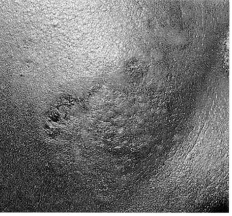

Figure 7-19   Discoid lupus erythematosus. This young woman was referred by her primary care physician for treatment-resistant eczema of the face.

antinuclear antibody (ANA) levels, Ro, La, liver and kidney enzyme levels, and urin-analysis.

Treatment

A broad-spectrum sunscreen and sun avoidance are crucial. A potent topical steroid may be tried initially. Intralesional steroids (e.g., triamcinolone, 5 to 10 mg/cc) are effective but risk atrophy. If topical or intralesional therapy fails, hydroxychloroquine or another antimalarial should be tried. Phenytoin (100 mg 3 times a day) provided excellent results in 88% of patients in one study. Prednisone, isotretinoin (e.g., 1 mg/kg/day), dapsone, thalidomide, methotrexate (e.g., given as for psoriasis), and azathioprine may be indicated.[11-13] Any hyperkeratotic nodules or growths should be evaluated for biopsy because SCCs have developed in chronic DLE lesions.

For children, topical steroids and sun protection are appropriate initial therapy. If needed, hydroxychloroquine may be given.[7]

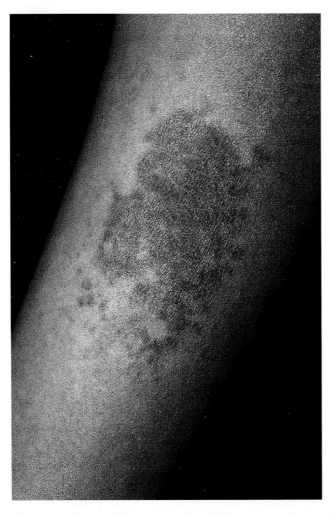

Figure 7-20 Cutaneous lupus erythematosus. An inflammatory plaque with significant postinflammatory hyperpigmentation developed on this woman's upper arm after several hours in the sun.

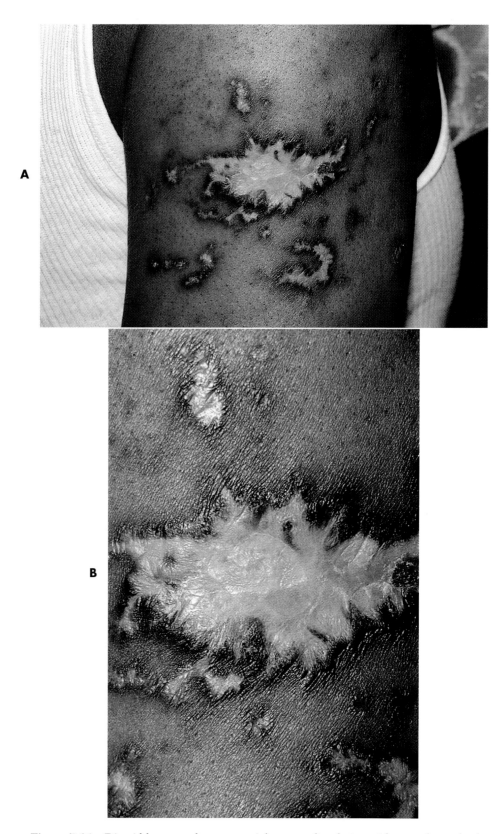

Figure 7-21   Discoid lupus erythematosus. A long-standing lesion with central atrophy, loss of pigmentation, and peripheral hyperpigmentation.

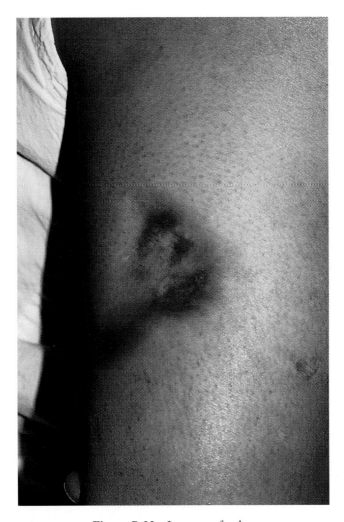

Figure 7-22   Lupus profundus.

Systemic Lupus Erythematosus

SLE is an autoimmune condition that affects multiple organ systems of the body. Making the diagnosis requires four of the following 11 criteria: malar rash, discoid rash, oral ulcers, photosensitivity, positive ANA, renal disease, neurologic disease, arthritis, serositis, hematologic disorders, or immunologic disorders. With regard to ethnicity, blacks seems to have SLE at a greater frequency and with greater severity than whites. For example, nephritis, pneumonitis, hypocomplementemia, and discoid lesions all are more common in blacks than in whites. Photosensitivity, in contrast, is found less commonly in blacks.[14] Black women seem to have an earlier onset of SLE and an earlier onset of nephritis.

Nephritis, pneumonitis, hypocomplementemia, and discoid lesions all are more common in blacks than in whites.

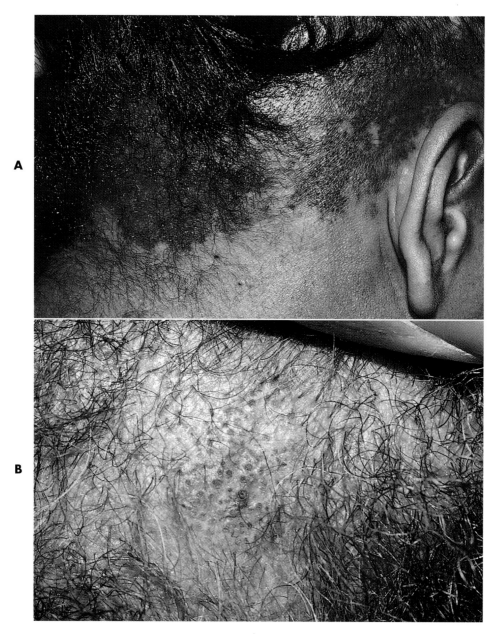

Figure 7-23 Discoid lupus erythematosus of the scalp. **A,** Alopecia and postinflammatory hyperpigmentation is shown. **B,** Multiple follicular plugs are seen.

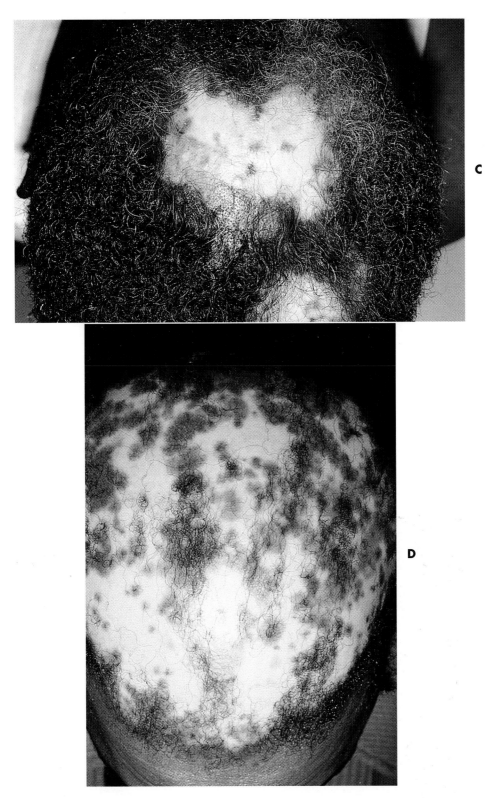

Figure 7-23, cont'd   Discoid lupus erythematosus of the scalp. **C,** A long-standing lesion. **D,** Widespread scarring alopecia. (Courtesy Michael O. Murphy, MD.)

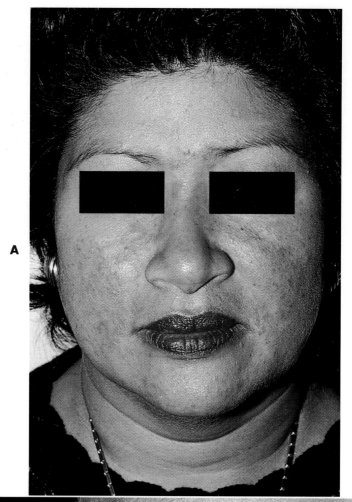

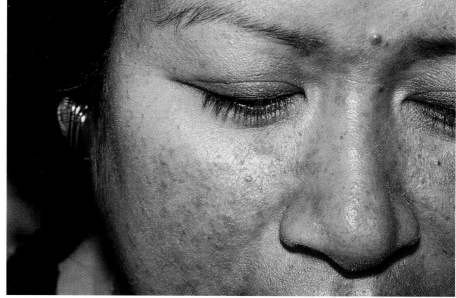

Figure 7-24   Ro-positive lupus erythematosus. A photoinduced rash in a young Hispanic woman positive for Ro (SS-A). She was ANA negative and had no other signs or symptoms of lupus erythematosus.

With regard to Asians, some studies have found that SLE may also occur more frequently in Asians than in whites. In Asian patients with SLE, there is a higher incidence (about 50%) of anti-Ro (SS-A) antibody positivity. Some of these patients have a peculiar annular erythema, but photosensitivity is less common.

In Asian patients with SLE, there is a higher incidence (about 50%) of anti-Ro (SS-A) antibody positivity. Some of these patients have a peculiar annular erythema, but photosensitivity is less common.

Clinical

Bilateral erythema of the cheeks and malar eminences (butterfly rash) or a more extensive photodistributed rash may be seen in patients with SLE (Figure 7-24). ANA is usually positive—often with a positive anti-dsDNA. Palmar erythema with tenderness is a common sign in black women, and it often signals a poor prognosis.

ANA-negative SLE does occur. These patients are often positive for ssDNA or Ro (SSA).

Treatment

With regard to the skin, if prednisone is needed for control of the rash, 20 to 30 mg/day is usually adequate for most patients. An antimalarial (e.g., hydroxychloroquine) is usually given as well. Once control is achieved, the prednisone may be tapered slowly (e.g., dropping 2.5 mg/month). Photoprotection is mandatory. Management of internal SLE manifestation is usually done in conjunction with a rheumatologist.

Other Connective Tissue Diseases

Morphea is rare in blacks, but systemic sclerosis does occur (Figure 7-25). A salt-and-pepper type of depigmentation is characteristic (Figure 7-26).

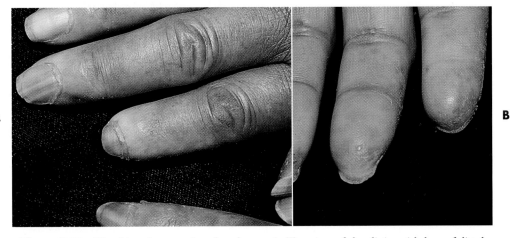

Figure 7-25 Hand involvement in scleroderma. **A,** Tapering of the digits with loss of distal tissue is seen. **B,** Note the pterygium inversus subunguis.

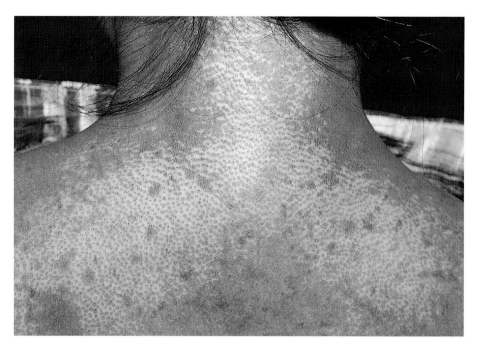

Figure 7-26   Salt-and-pepper depigmentation in scleroderma.

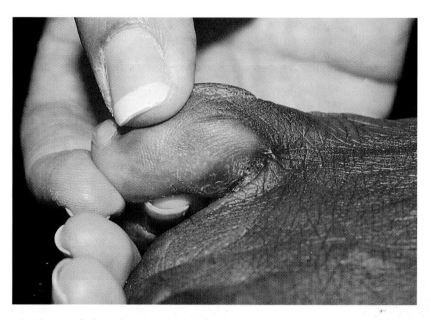

Figure 7-27   A soft, hyperkeratotic nodule (corn) is found on the medial aspect of the fifth toe.

CORNS

Corns result from constant pressure at that site, often caused by an underlying bony prominence or exostosis. A hyperkeratotic, painful papule on the sole, dorsa of the toes, or in the web spaces (Figure 7-27) is characteristic. Paring reveals the characteristic translucent core of a corn; this is in contrast to a verruca, which reveals black dots and bleeding. Pain is immediately relieved by paring, which may be done initially in the office and subsequently by the patient. A salicylic acid plaster may soften the corn. Donut-shaped pads and different footwear can relieve the pressure. Ultimately, surgery may be performed to remove an underlying exostosis if present.

CUTANEOUS T-CELL LYMPHOMA

Cutaneous T-cell lymphoma in dark-skinned patients may take the typical form of scaly areas, plaques (Figure 7-28, *A*), nodules, or tumors. Rarely, cutaneous T-cell lymphoma may present with purely macular, hypopigmented lesions[15-17] (Figure 7-28, *B*). The lesions may be smooth or slightly scaly and either normal to palpation or slightly indurated. Children may be affected, and some have been initially misdiagnosed as having pityriasis alba. PUVA has been a successful treatment. Repigmentation may occur.

CUTIS VERTICIS GYRATA

"Meaty" gyrate folds of the scalp in a young man are most characteristic of cutis verticis gyrata (Figure 7-29). It usually occurs as an isolated finding but may be a component of pachydermoperiostosis (Figure 7-30), in which the face also becomes thickened and develops deep folds and furrows. Clubbing of the fingers, oiliness of the face, and palmarplantar hyperhidrosis may occur. Cosmetic surgery to debulk the excess tissue may be beneficial.

DERMATITIS CRURIS PUSTULOSA ET ATROPHICANS

Dermatitis cruris pustulosa et atrophicans is a rare condition of the shins of darker-skinned patients. The skin is atrophic, shiny, and studded with follicular pustules (Figure 7-31). Staphylococcus is often cultured. It is presumed that the constant application of various oils contributes to this condition. Treating any infection with oral antibiotics and stopping any topical emollients usually results in significant improvement.

DERMATOFIBROMA

A firm, dark brown, velvety papule or plaque that dimples in the center with lateral pressure is characteristic of a dermatofibroma in a black person (Figure 7-32). The leg is the favored site, but it may occur on the upper back or elsewhere (Figure 7-33). Multiple dermatofibromas (e.g., more than 15) have been associated with various diseases, including LE and scleroderma.

No treatment is needed. A shave excision may help if the lesion is raised. Elliptical excision usually leaves a scar whose appearance is worse than that of the original lesion. Cryotherapy should not be used in the darker-skinned patient.

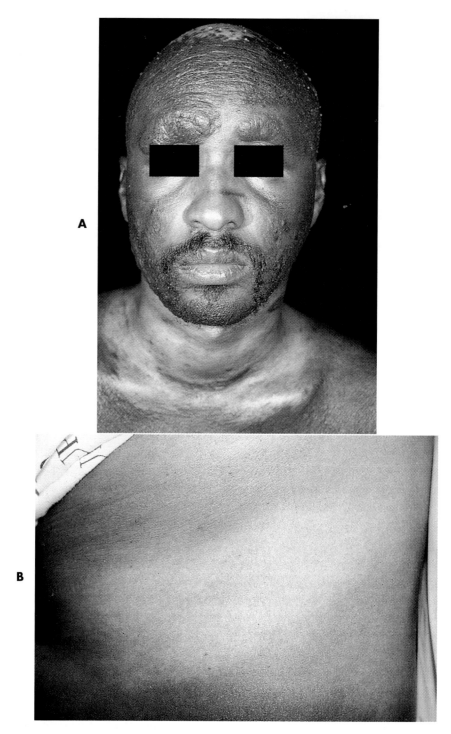

Figure 7-28   Cutaneous T-cell lymphoma with hypopigmentation. (Courtesy Stuart Lessin, Associate Professor of Dermatology, University of Pennsylvania School of Medicine.)

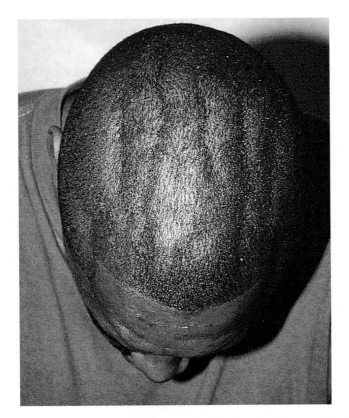

Figure 7-29 Cutis verticis gyrata is an isolated finding in this young black man.

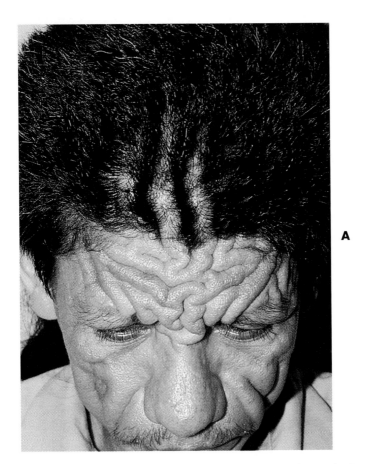

A

Figure 7-30 Pachydermoperiostosis in a young Hispanic man. Note the cerebriform folding of the forehead **(A).**

Continued

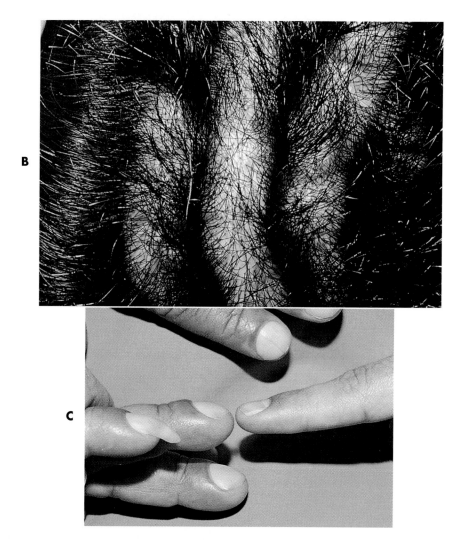

Figure 7-30, cont'd   Pachydermoperiostosis in a young Hispanic man. Note the cerebriform folding of the scalp **(B)** and the clubbing (normal finger on the right) **(C)**.

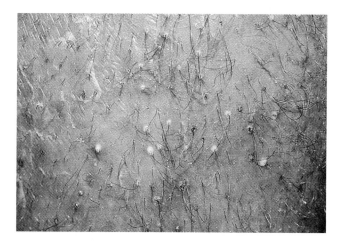

Figure 7-31   Dermatitis cruris pustulosa et atrophicans.

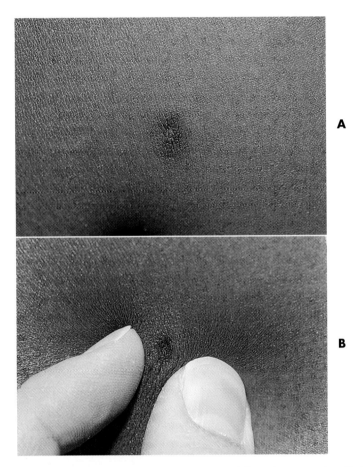

A

B

Figure 7-32   Dermatofibroma. Dimpling in the center with lateral pressure is called the *buttonhole sign.*

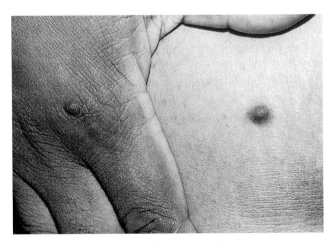

Figure 7-33   Two dermatofibromas.

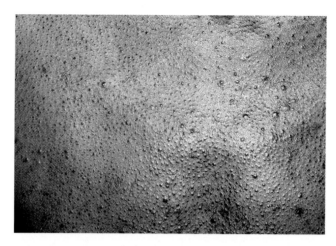

Figure 7-34   Disseminate and recurrent infundibulofolliculitis in a young man.

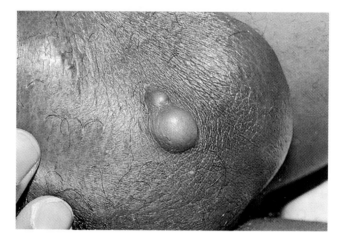

Figure 7-35   Epidermal inclusion cyst. Two are seen here on the scrotum.

DISSEMINATE AND RECURRENT INFUNDIBULOFOLLICULITIS

Disseminate and recurrent infundibulofolliculitis is seen primarily in black adults.[18] Clinically, hundreds of uniform, 1 to 2 mm, pruritic, follicular papules will be visible on the trunk (Figure 7-34). The neck, arms, and buttocks may also be affected. The condition may last for years, even decades. Histologically, there is a mixed infiltrate and spongiosis of the infundibulum of affected hair follicles. This condition has been thought to represent a variant of follicular eczema, but many of the reported patients have not had a personal or family history of atopy. A topical steroid may be tried but is often ineffective.

EPIDERMAL INCLUSION CYST

The epidermal inclusion cyst presents as a dermal nodule within the skin (Figure 7-35). In a white person, the lesion may often take on a whitish color, or if the keratin

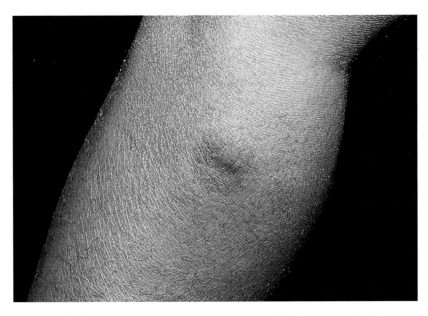

Figure 7-36 Postinflammatory hyperpigmentation at the site of a fixed drug eruption 2 weeks prior.

has oxidized, a dark brown or black color. In the darker-skinned patient, these color changes are obscured. A pore is usually visible and an unpleasant-smelling white material may periodically drain from it. A lipoma can be distinguished from an epidermal inclusion cyst because it lies below the skin and no pore is visible. If bothersome, epidermal inclusion cysts can be surgically removed in their entirety. Draining the lesion leaves the cyst wall intact and guarantees a recurrence.

FIXED DRUG ERUPTION

Single or multiple, dusky-red, round or oval lesions occurring repeatedly in a fixed site after each exposure to the offending drug are characteristic of a fixed drug eruption. In the dark-skinned patient, a jet-black color is typical. With each subsequent exposure to the drug, the initial lesion may increase in size, and additional lesions may develop. A hyperpigmented patch is often left that fades over months (Figure 7-36). The history is usually sufficient for diagnosis. Oral challenge can confirm the diagnosis, but runs the rare risk of anaphylaxis. Typical drugs to consider include tetracycline, sulfa drugs, ampicillin, and phenolphthalein. In children, inquire about acetaminophen, ASA, ipecac, and phenolphthalein use. Usually no treatment is needed for the acute outbreak other than identifying the offending drug and avoiding future exposure.

FOLLICULAR OCCLUSION TRIAD

The follicular occlusion triad is made up of three diseases that often occur together: hidradenitis suppurativa, acne conglobata, and dissecting cellulitis of the scalp.

Hidradenitis suppurativa appears to be a process of poral occlusion of the pilosebaceous unit with secondary inflammation of the apocrine glands. Inflammatory nodules and sterile abscesses develop initially in the axilla (Figure 7-37), the groin, the inframammary area, and/or the perianal area. With chronic inflammation, sinus tracts, fistulas, and hypertrophic scarring develop. Medical treatment usually takes the form of weight loss if overweight, reduction of friction by the avoidance of heat and tight-fitting clothing, and the use of powders. For early, inflammatory, but sterile lesions, triamcinolone 2.5 to 5 mg/ml may be injected intralesionally. Incision and drainage may be done if the lesion is fluctuant, but this procedure may contribute to the scarring. Once lesions have become chronic, and especially if drainage is present, antibiotics, either topical (e.g., clindamycin) or oral, are helpful. Exteriorization of chronically draining sinuses may be necessary. For definitive cure, wide surgical excision with heal-

---

Hidradenitis suppurativa appears to be a process of poral occlusion of the pilosebaceous unit with secondary inflammation of the apocrine glands.

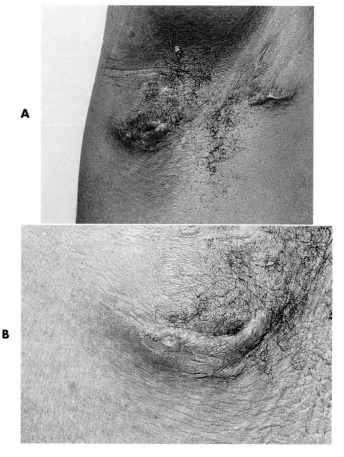

Figure 7-37 Hidradenitis suppurativa. Multiple inflammatory nodules are seen, some with draining sinuses. Note the scars of partial excisions that, in general, improve the condition temporarily, but don't cure the problem.

ing by secondary intention should be done, preferably by someone with experience in this area. Narrow excision of inflamed areas may help temporarily but has a high recurrence rate.

The patient with *acne conglobata* is affected with multiple comedones, inflammatory nodules with pus, scarring, and sinus tracts of the back, buttocks, face (Figure 7-38), and chest. The lesion characteristic of this disease is the larger comedone with multiple openings. Treatment often consists of chronic oral antibiotics (e.g., tetracycline 500 mg twice daily, minocycline 100 mg twice daily). A course of isotretinoin is recommended by many, but the drug is not as effective as it is against acne vulgaris. Incision and drainage of acutely inflamed or fluctuant areas may be necessary. Chronically draining sinus tracts may need to be externalized.

The patient with *dissecting cellulitis of the scalp* (also known as *perifolliculitis capitis abscedens et suffodiens*) is plagued by inflammatory nodules, sinus tracts, chronic drainage, crusting alopecia, and scarring (Figure 7-39). Bacterial cultures should be taken and *Staphylococcus aureus* is often found. Indeed, darker-skinned patients who use abundant hair oils are predisposed to bacterial infections of the scalp (unassociated with dissecting cellulitis of the scalp). It is only when inflammatory lesions continue to appear despite repeatedly negative cultures and multiple courses of oral antibiotics that the diagnosis of dissecting cellulitis of the scalp is confirmed. Intralesional triamcinolone and isotretinoin, marsupialization of the sinus tracts, or incision and drainage of abscesses are also treatment options.

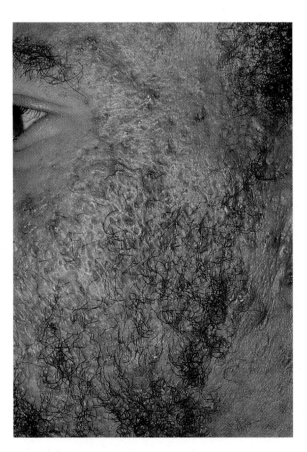

Figure 7-38   Acne conglobata.

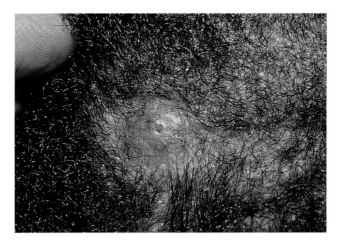

Figure 7-39   Dissecting cellulitis of the scalp. Inflammatory nodules, sinus tracts, chronic drainage, crusting alopecia, and scarring occur in this disease, which is also known as *perifolliculitis capitis abscedens et suffodiens*.

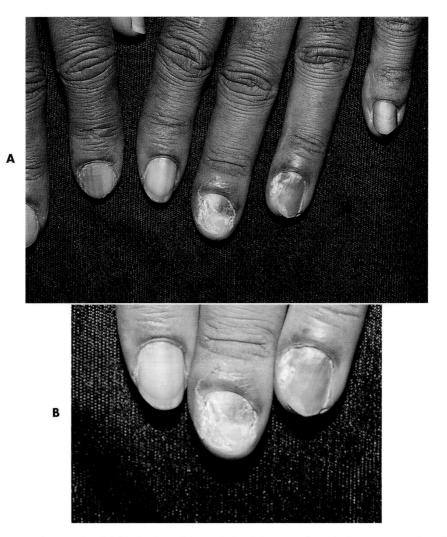

Figure 7-40   Candidal infection of the nail. *Candidas tropicalis* and *albicans* were cultured.

FUNGAL INFECTIONS

Onychomycosis

Clinical

Onychomycosis is common in all races. The most common clinical presentations include separation of the nail plate and bed (onycholysis) and accumulation of subungual debris. The entire nail may be progressively destroyed. The causative organism may be a dermatophyte, yeast (e.g., candida [Figure 7-40]), or a mold.

Topical antifungal agents are usually ineffective. Oral therapy is needed. The patient should be informed of the low but potential risks associated with oral therapy, after which he or she may decline treatment. Terbinafine, itraconazole, or fluconazole are effective treatments.

Tinea Corporis

The erythema may be masked in tinea corporis, but the abundant scaly appearance remains (Figures 7-41 and 7-42). A topical antifungal agent is effective for localized disease. An oral antifungal agent (e.g., griseofulvin) is best for disseminated disease. If onychomycosis causes frequent recurrences, the nails should be cleared as well with terbinafine or itraconazole.

Tinea Cruris

Red, scaly plaques radiating out from the inguinal fold onto the inner thigh are characteristic of tinea cruruis. In darker-skinned patients, the erythema is often undistinguishable (Figure 7-43). The border is usually scaly, raised, and KOH positive. Itching may vary from absent to severe. A topical antifungal is usually curative, although an oral antifungal may be given in extensive or resistant cases. The topical antifungal

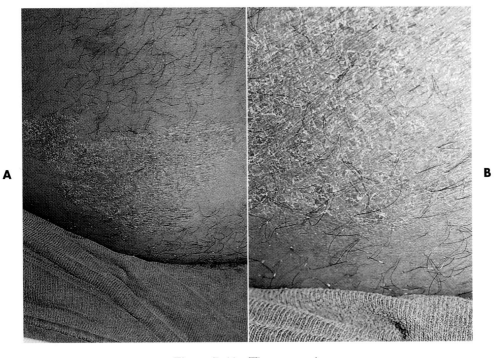

A   **B**

Figure 7-41   Tinea corporis.

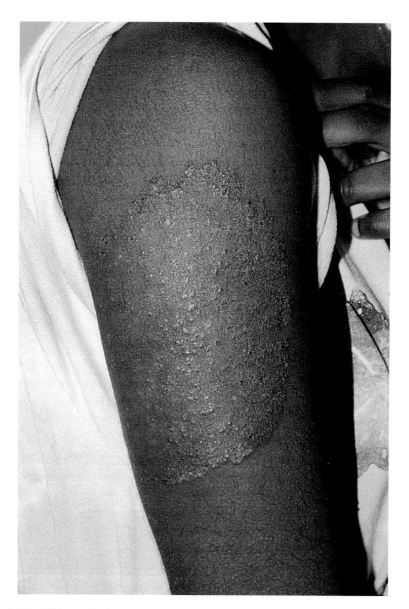

Figure 7-42   This patch of tinea corporis was incorrectly treated as eczema with a potent topical steroid.

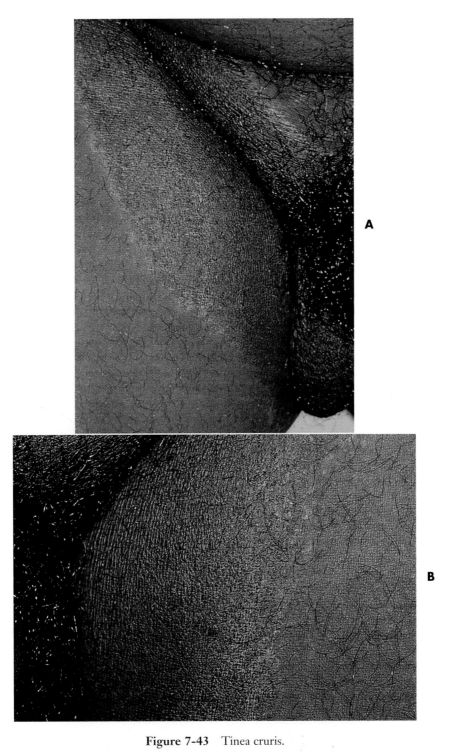

Figure 7-43   Tinea cruris.

should also be applied to the feet on a long-term basis because tinea pedis is invariably present and a source of recurrent infection.

Tinea Faciei

A dermatophyte infection may occasionally involve the face. It usually presents as an annular, raised arc or plaque with variable scale (Figure 7-44).

Tinea Pedis

Scaling of the web spaces only or of the entire sole (moccasin distribution) may occur in tinea pedis. KOH examination or culture is confirmatory. Rarely, the inflammation can be so severe that it causes bulla formation (Figure 7-45).

Tinea Versicolor

Clinical

Tinea versicolor is a common condition caused by the fungal organism Pityrosporum. Hypopigmented or hyperpigmented patches result from the body's response to this organism and its metabolic products. Blacks are commonly affected, probably because any pigmentary changes are quite noticeable and possibly because of their increased rate of sweating.

Hypopigmented (Figure 7-46) or hyperpigmented (Figure 7-47) patches on the trunk and/or arms of a young adult that have a slight scale when scraped (Figure 7-48) are characteristic. Lesions may also occur on the arms (Figure 7-49). Hypopigmented, slightly scaly lesions may occur on the face (Figure 7-50). Large, dark areas; uniformly light areas; or coalescent, perifollicular, hypopigmented macules may be prominent.

A KOH preparation showing spaghetti-and-meatball hyphal forms is diagnostic (Figure 7-51).

Text continued on p. 83

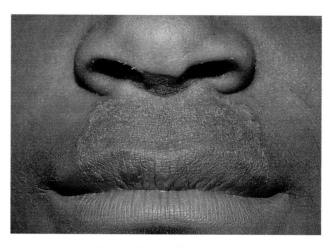

Figure 7-44 Tinea faciei.

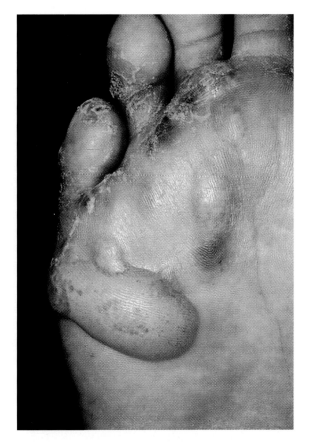

Figure 7-45   Bullous tinea.

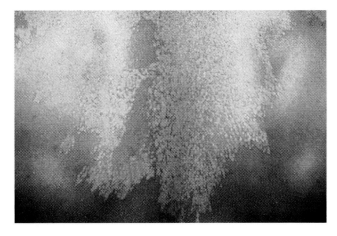

Figure 7-46   Tinea versicolor with coalescent hypopigmented macules.

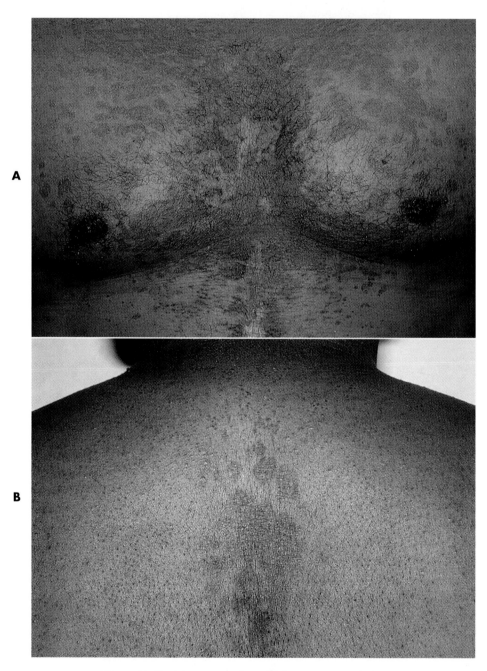

Figure 7-47 Tinea versicolor with hyperpigmented plaques.

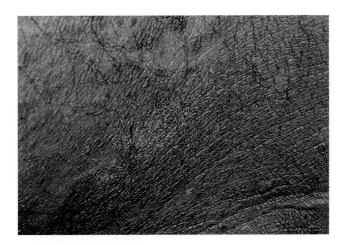

Figure 7-48   Tinea versicolor. Note the slight scale when scratched.

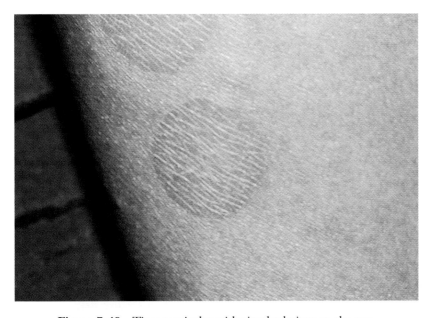

Figure 7-49   Tinea versicolor with circular lesions on the arm.

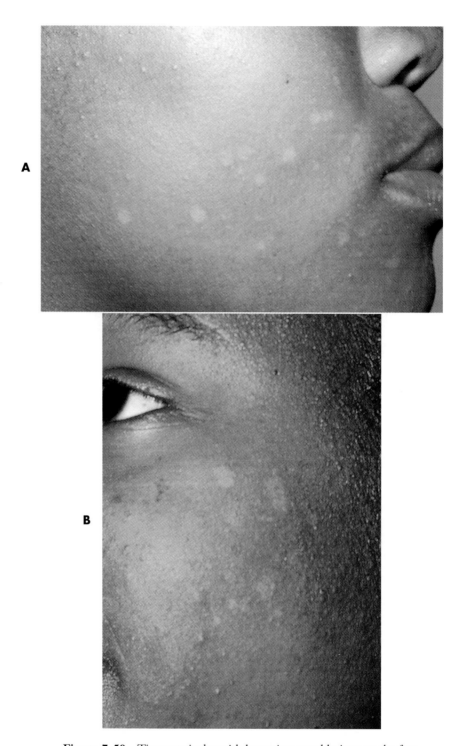

Figure 7-50 Tinea versicolor with hypopigmented lesions on the face.

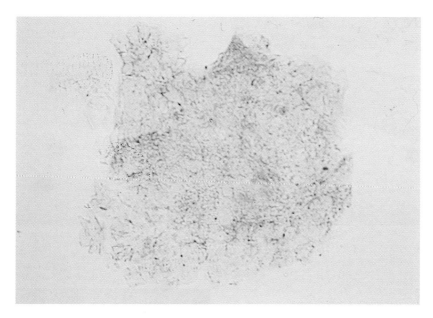

Figure 7-51 Tinea versicolor with spaghetti-and-meatball forms on KOH. (Courtesy Terence C. O'Grady, MD.)

Treatment

The Pityrosporum must be killed, or more accurately, its numbers kept to a minimum to facilitate resolution of the lesions and allow the pigmentation to normalize. Selenium sulfide 2.5% or ketoconazole shampoo used to lather the scalp and trunk for 5 to 10 minutes a day for 1 week followed by reduction in the frequency of use is one successful approach to therapy. Alternatives include oral ketoconazole (e.g., two doses of 400 mg separated by 7 days or 200 mg every day for 2 weeks) or fluconazole (e.g., 400 mg as a single dose). Long-term prophylactic treatment (e.g., use of one of the above shampoos every 2 weeks) prevents recurrences, which are otherwise common. Ketoconazole 400 mg orally every 14 days has been used as a prophylactic intervention without adverse laboratory effects.

GRANULOMA ANNULARE

Granuloma annulare is a relatively common condition caused by an "immune attack" of the dermis. It presents with palpable, dermal, nonscaly papules and/or nodules (Figure 7-52). The lesions tend to spread out from a central focus, often resulting in annular lesions. The fingers, dorsa of the hands, and elbows are common sites. Disseminated forms occur. Treatment is not needed, but intralesional steroid injection may be tried. The usual precautions must be taken, given the risk of hypopigmentation.

HIV INFECTION

Immunosuppression can predispose to a variety of conditions including Kaposi's sarcoma (Figure 7-53) and chronic herpes simplex infection (Figure 7-54).

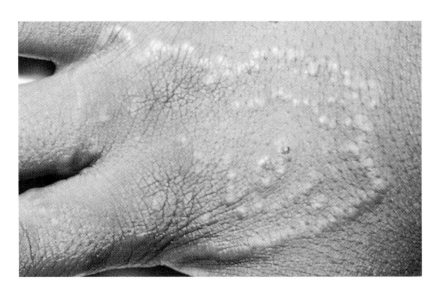

Figure 7-52 Granuloma annulare.

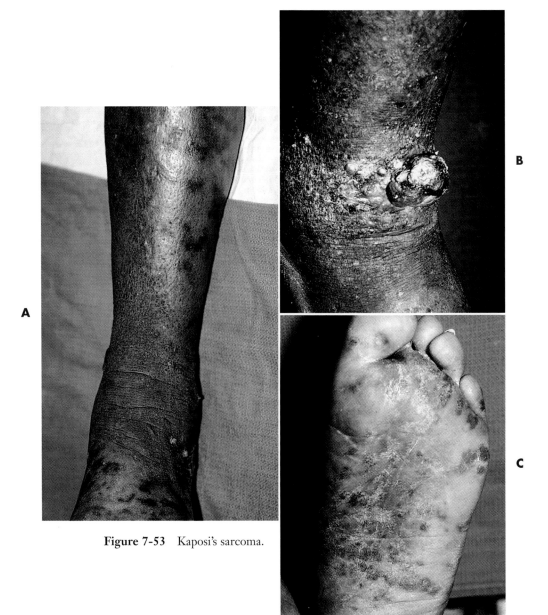

Figure 7-53 Kaposi's sarcoma.

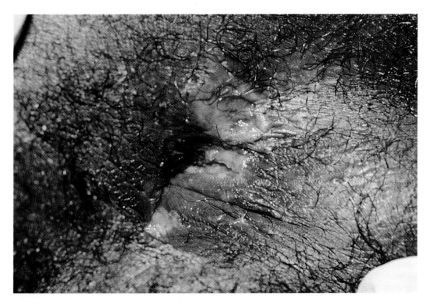

Figure 7-54 Chronic herpes simplex infection in the perianal area. A chronic ulcer in the perianal area of an HIV-positive patient represents herpes until proved otherwise.

HYPERSENSITIVITY SYNDROME

A diffuse maculopapular eruption along with fever, lymphadenopathy, and hepatitis 4 weeks to 3 months after starting an anticonvulsant such as phenytoin, carbamazepine, primidone, or phenobarbitol is characteristic of hypersensitivity syndrome (HS) (Figure 7-55). Some reports have stated that this condition is more common in the black patient. Drugs other than anticonvulsants may cause this hypersensitivity syndrome and include allopurinol, atenolol, captopril, chlorpropamide, dapsone, diltiazem, isoniazid, mexiletine, minocycline, phenylbutazone, and sulfasalazine.[19,20] Follicular pustules,[21] erythema multiforme (EM), or toxic epidermal necrolysis (TEN) may occur instead of the maculopapular rash. Other common findings include mucosal inflammation and crusting as in Stevens-Johnson syndrome (SJS), facial edema, and conjunctivitis (with possible scarring and synechia). Some would say that if there is significant mucosal inflammation and crusting, the diagnosis is SJS. If there is only aphthoid ulceration, pharyngitis, or conjunctivitis with the other typical findings of HS, then HS is the diagnosis.

Etiology

There is some evidence that affected patients who have taken anticonvulsants are unable to detoxify arene oxide.[22] However, other patients[23] have been found to be allergic to the medications.

Systemic

Severe liver dysfunction is typical, and renal and pulmonary compromise may occur. Leukocytosis with eosinophilia occurs. Hepatic necrosis and death are possible.

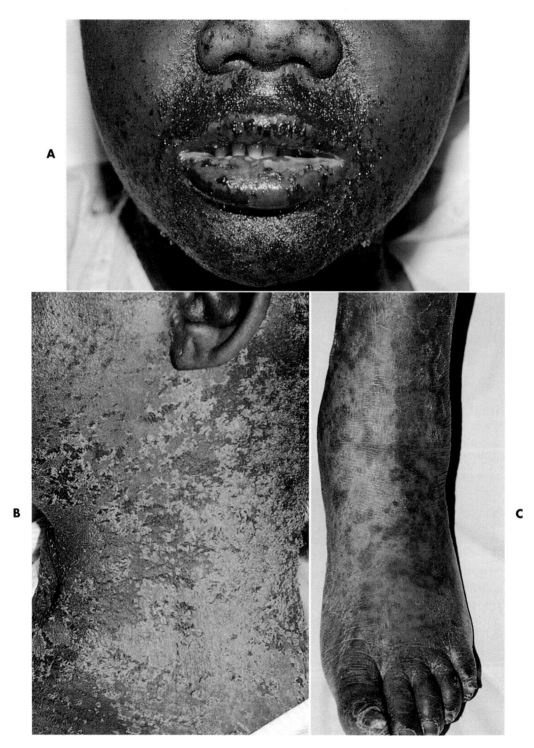

Figure 7-55   Hypersensitivity syndrome caused by Dilantin.

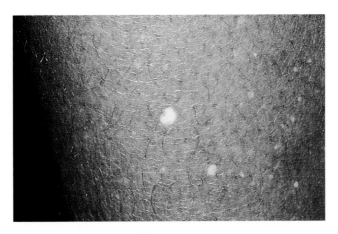

Figure 7-56   Idiopathic guttate hypomelanosis.

Differential Diagnosis

The patient with the classic drug eruption does not have fever, myalgias, and hepatitis. SJS may be hard to differentiate if there is mucocutaneous involvement. Patients with drug-induced pseudolymphoma have more subacute papulonodular or infiltrated plaques, without visceral involvement. A biopsy of the skin also shows a dense lymphocytic infiltrate mimicking lymphoma.

Treatment

The offending drug should be stopped immediately. Prednisone instituted as early as possible has been recommended.[24] Valproate sodium appears to be tolerated in patients with this syndrome secondary to anticonvulsants.

IDIOPATHIC GUTTATE HYPOMELANOSIS

Idiopathic guttate hypomelanosis occurs in all races, but is particularly noticeable in those with darker skin. Multiple white macules, usually 1 to 4 mm in diameter and symmetrically distributed on the outer forearms or extensor legs, are characteristic (Figure 7-56). Women are more commonly affected than men, especially those women over 40 years of age. Patients should be reassured that these lesions are benign, tend to stay small, and do not represent vitiligo.

INTERTRIGO

Clinical

A moist, red, often macerated rash in the intertriginous folds of the groin in an obese man is characteristic of intertrigo (Figure 7-57). Because of increased heat and sweating, the rash is usually worse during the summer. Intertrigo may also occur under pendulous breasts, in the gluteal cleft, in the abdominal folds of the very obese, in the finger or toe webs, or even in the folds extending from the corners of the mouth in perlèche. Intertrigo may develop in any place where the skin does not stay cool and dry.

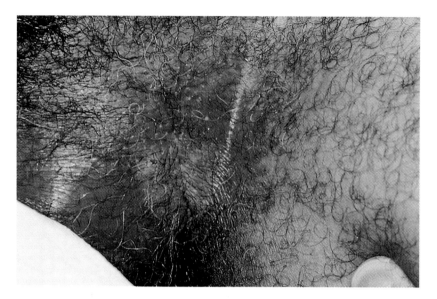

Figure 7-57   Intertrigo.

Diagnosis

The diagnosis of intertrigo is one of exclusion. One must always consider tinea, inverse psoriasis, or candidiasis. A negative KOH preparation helps exclude *Candida* and dermatophyte. Seborrheic dermatitis of the folds may be a consideration; in fact, moist, erythematous patches in the folds may present a diagnostic conundrum.

Treatment

The affected area should be kept cool and dry. After showering, the area may be dried with a blow dryer. Superabsorbent powders are also helpful in this regard (e.g., Zeasorb or Zeasorb AF). A mild topical steroid solution or cream may be soothing and antipruritic. Ointments should be avoided. Some patients sweat at night, and the bedroom should be cooled sufficiently to prevent this. Sweating is permitted during exercise, but friction should be minimized, and patients should shower immediately after. Patients should be told to be aware of the "sweatiness" of the affected area and to make sure it stays cool and dry at all times, except during exercise.

LICHEN PLANUS

Clinical

Lichen planus usually presents purple, polygonal, flat-topped papules in white skin. The color of the papule is modified in black skin. Purple, brown, or black are more typical colors. Postinflammatory hyperpigmentation is usually quite prominent and persistent. Some have thought that lichen planus, when it occurs in blacks, is more widespread and severe as a rule, but this remains to be proved. Common sites of involvement are the inner wrists (Figure 7-58), the penis, and the oral mucosa. Hypertrophic (Figure 7-59) and annular (Figures 7-60 and 7-61) forms occur. A white, lacelike appearance of the surface (Wickham's striae) is characteristic and is often quite prominently visible on the oral mucosa of a black person (Figures 7-62 to 7-64).

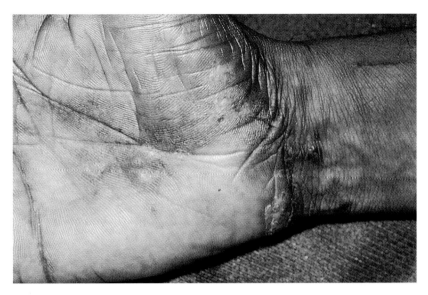

Figure 7-58   A characteristic lichen planus site. Note how dark the lesions are.

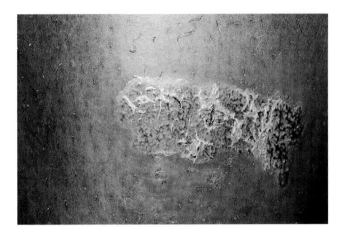

Figure 7-59   Hypertrophic lichen planus of the leg. Note the reticulate surface.

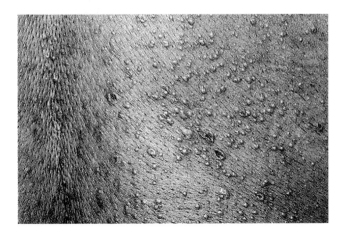

Figure 7-60   Early lichen planus with papules and annular forms.

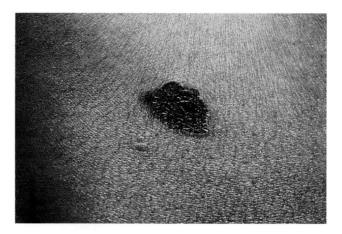

Figure 7-61 Annular lichen planus lesions with a characteristic pigmented center.

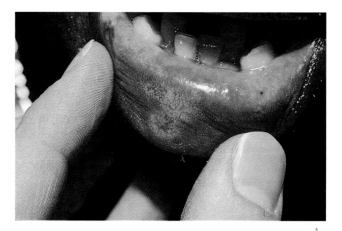

Figure 7-62 Lichen planus of the lip. Note the prominent Wickham's striae.

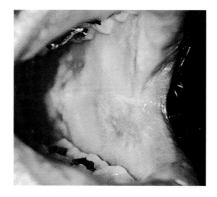

Figure 7-63 Lichen planus of the buccal mucosa.

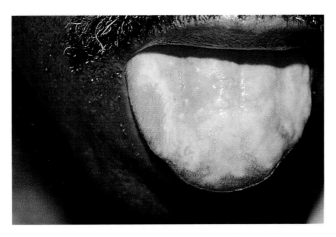

Figure 7-64   Lichen planus of the tongue. Note the annular morphology.

Patients with chronic liver disease (e.g., primary biliary cirrhosis, chronic active hepatitis) have twice the risk of developing lichen planus compared with the general population. Some of these patients are infected with hepatitis B and some with hepatitus C.

Treatment

For limited disease, a potent topical steroid ointment should be tried, and the patient should be admonished not to scratch. The patient should also be cautioned about potential hypopigmentation of the surrounding normal skin. A steroid-impregnated tape, changed daily, may also help. Systemic corticosteroids (e.g., prednisone 40 to 60 mg/day tapered over 4 to 6 weeks or intramuscular triamcinolone 40 to 60 mg) are quite effective and often needed, but recurrences are common so their use should be tapered slowly over months.

MELANOCYTIC NEVI

Clinical

Both black children and black adults may develop melanocytic nevi (Figure 7-65), although they occur in much fewer numbers in blacks than in whites. For example, Kopf et al[25] studied the incidence of melanocytic nevi on the lateral and medial aspects of the arms of both whites and blacks. They found an equal number of nevi on the medial and lateral aspects of the arms of black patients (5.5%). In contrast, 24.5% of white patients had nevi on the lateral aspect of the arms and 11.1% had nevi on the medial aspect of the arms. Kopf et al wondered if increased sun exposure was the reason for more nevi laterally in white patients. This would be consistent with a finding of fewer nevi in black patients because their melanin composition greatly decreases the amount of UV light that reaches the dermal epidermal junction.

Any pigmented lesion should be evaluated by the ABCD criteria (**A**symmetric shape, irregular **B**order, multiple **C**olors, **D**iameter 7 mm or greater). If two or more

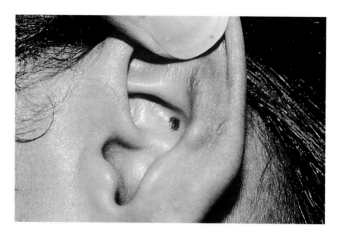

Figure 7-65   Acquired melanocytic nevus.

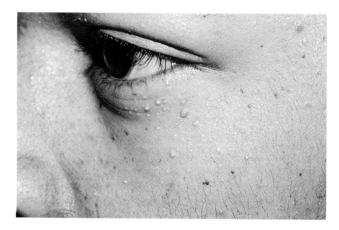

Figure 7-66   Multiple milia are seen in the periorbital area. A few lesions of dermatosis papulosa nigra are seen as well.

of the criteria are present, the lesion should be removed in its entirety. For a more thorough discussion of melanoma in blacks, see Chapter 3.

MILIA

Milia represent tiny epidermal inclusion cysts. Clinically, they appear as tiny, whitish papules on the face, usually about the eyes (Figure 7-66).

PERFORATING DISORDER OF DIALYSIS

Pruritic, dome-shaped papules occur on the extremities of patients on dialysis (Figure 7-67). Histologic examination shows perforation of both collagen and elastin.

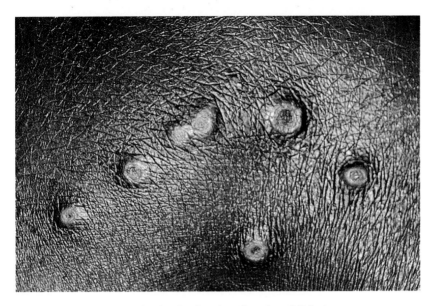

Figure 7-67   Perforating disorder of dialysis.

PEMPHIGUS FOLIACEUS

Clinical

Erosions, bullae, and crusted plaques affect the face (Figure 7-68), chest, and elsewhere in pemphigus foliaceus. Some patients may have their disease exacerbated by UV exposure. Direct immunofluorescence (DIF) shows intercellular IgG and/or C3. Histologically, the separation occurs high in the epidermis. An endemic type also known as *fogo selvagem* occurs primarily in Brazil and mainly affects children and young adults.

PITYRIASIS ROSEA

In blacks, the percent of total visits to a skin clinic for pityriasis rosea ranges from 0.5% to 2.5%.[26] In the classic form, a herald patch appears first, followed 1 to 3 weeks later by an oval, papulosquamous eruption running parallel to cleavage lines on the trunk, neck, groin, and proximal extremities (Figures 7-69 and 7-70).

Does pityriasis rosea appear differently in blacks? It is clear that the erythema or rosy color is not apparent in blacks, and thus the term *pityriasis rosea* is not very descriptive.[27] It has also been suggested that a papular pattern often predominates in blacks, in which both follicular and nonfollicular papules are distributed on the trunk and proximal extremities. This pattern is certainly present early in the disease, but it is unclear what percentage of the time this form is the predominant morphology in well-developed cases. For example, in Ahmed's report of 81 patients from the Sudan[24] with pityriasis rosea, 68 had the typical oval, papulosquamous pattern. A few had patterns that were circinate or psoriasiform, but no vesicular or purely papular variants were reported. Of note, in 10 of the 81 cases, the condition was more prominant distally than centrally. Inverse pityriasis rosea may be more frequent in black skin, where the lesions begin in the axillae and groin and then spread centrally.

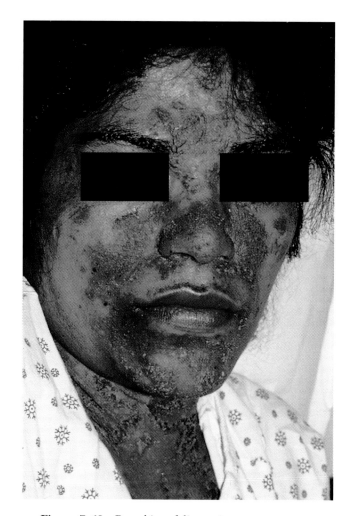

Figure 7-68   Pemphigus foliaceus in a young woman.

Figure 7-69   Early pityriasis rosea, where the predominant lesion is an erythematous papule. Within a week, the more typical papulosquamous plaques had formed.

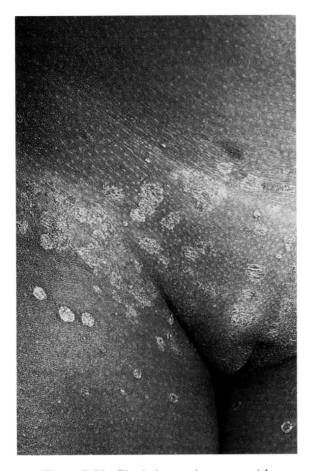

Figure 7-70   Pityriasis rosea in a young girl.

No treatment is necessary because the disease tends to run a benign course over 6 to 9 weeks. Topical steroids may be given for pruritus. In severe cases, UVB may be given.

PITYRIASIS ROTUNDA

Clinical

Multiple, strikingly circular, scaly, ichthyosiform lesions are characteristic of pityriasis rotunda. These lesions are associated with malignancy (e.g., hepatocellular carcinoma; carcinoma of the esophagus, stomach, or prostate; chronic lymphocytic leukemia [CLL]; myeloma) and clear when the neoplasm is treated. Pityriasis rotunda has been reported more commonly in Asian and black patients but can occur in whites, where there does not as yet seem to be an association with malignancy.[28] The course of the disease is chronic, lasting many years.

Other patients have had concurrent tuberculosis, HIV, and trypanosomiasis. The common thread may be chronic systemic disease and weight loss.

Treatment

When associated with malignancy or internal disease, treatment of that disease and improvement of the functional and nutritional status of the patient often clears

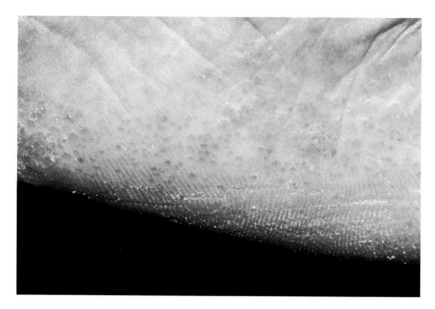

Figure 7-71   Deep-seated "tapioca" vesicles of pompholyx on the sides of the feet.

the pityriasis rotunda. Anecdotal success of treatment with 10% lactic acid lotion, etretinate, and vitamin A has been reported.

POMPHOLYX

Clinical

Tiny "tapioca" vesicles of the sides of the fingers, fingertips, palms, and soles (Figure 7-71) occur in this syndrome, which is also called *dyshidrotic eczema*. The affected areas may become red, scaly, and weepy, and the patient usually complains of intense itching.

Diagnosis

The most important clinical distinction is between pompholyx and irritant contact dermatitis (ICD). Admittedly, many patients have both conditions; but in terms of treatment, the eczematous areas of ICD need emollients and protection from irritants. The deep-seated, very itchy blisters of pompholyx need potent topical steroids.

Treatment

The physician should always try to determine with the patient any trigger factors. Does contact with chemicals, friction, or specific items cause the breakout? Usually no triggers are found, but this exercise is always important. High-potency topical steroids are the mainstay of treament. Lidex, Valisone, Diprosone, or even a class I ointment at bedtime or twice daily are usually needed. These should be applied on the volar surface. Long-term application on the dorsal surface may cause atrophy and, in dark-skinned patients, hypopigmentation. When there is more scale than erythema, keratolytics may be prescribed (e.g., LacHydrin lotion 12%).

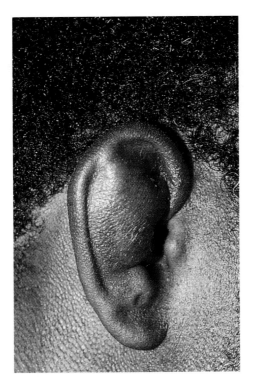

Figure 7-72   Pseudocyst of the ear.

PSEUDOCYST

A pseudocyst appears as a nontender, firm, intracartilaginous, cystic lesion of the ear (Figure 7-72). It may be preceded by trauma (as occurred in two boys after ear pulling for their birthday) or in association with atopic dermatitis. Drainage yields a thick, viscous fluid. Several successful approaches to therapy have been reported. After drainage, a sclerosing agent may be instilled and bolstering sutures placed. Alternatively, the anterior cartilaginous wall may be removed. Simple aspiration usually leads to recurrence.

PSORIASIS

Studies do not agree on the exact incidence of psoriasis in blacks (Figures 7-73 to 7-78), although it seems to be only slightly less common than in whites. In one study, 44 out of 5250 (0.8%) patients seen in a Nigerian skin clinic had psoriasis.[29] Guttate, plaque-type, and erythrodermic forms all occur. The typical ham-colored erythema is obscured in blacks. Localization of lesions, scale, and the uniformly raised nature of the plaques allows the diagnosis.

A potent topical steroid, with the usual caution about atrophy and hypopigmentation, may be used initially. Calcipotriene, tazarotene, tars, and anthralin are alternatives. Methotrexate, PUVA, UVB, and acitretin are appropriate therapy for more severe disease.

Text continued on p. 102

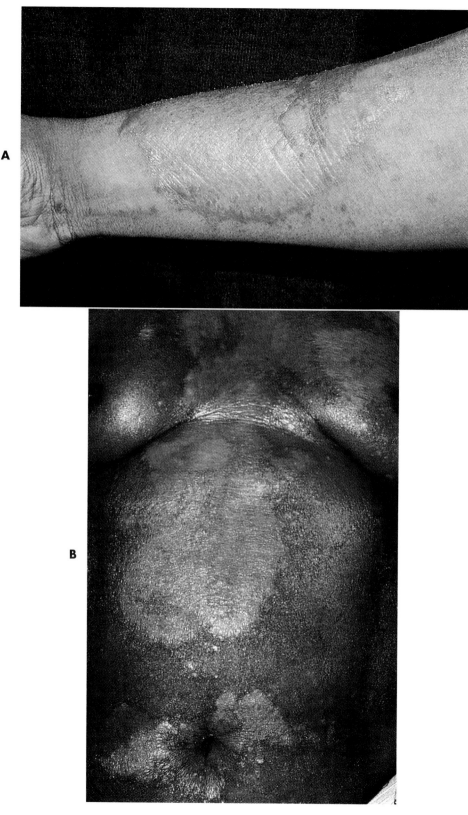

Figure 7-73   Chronic plaque type of psoriasis.

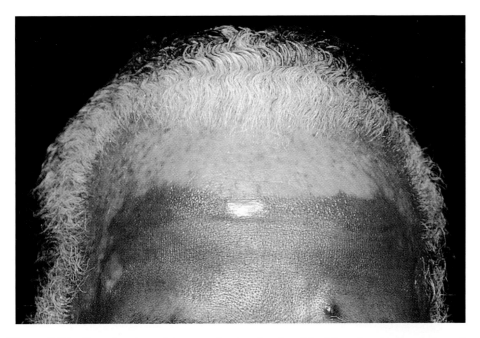

Figure 7-74   Complete loss of pigmentation has developed in this patient in a band about the hairline where his psoriasis commonly occurred.

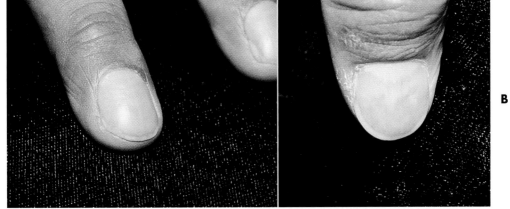

Figure 7-75   Nail psoriasis. **A,** Pits are seen. **B,** Nail bed involvement causes these "oil spots."

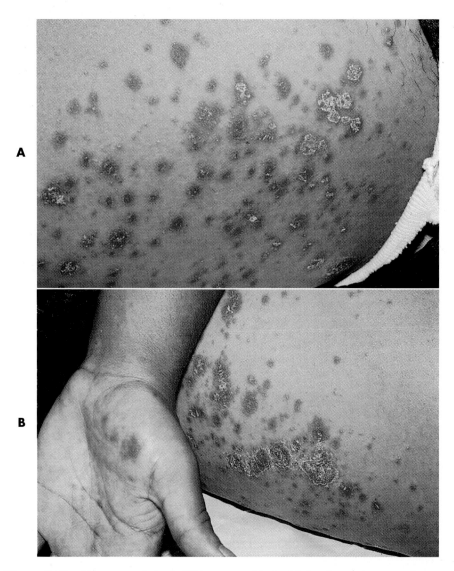

Figure 7-76   Guttate psoriasis. **A,** This teenage black girl developed these papulosquamous plaques over several weeks. **B,** Involvement of the palms made secondary syphilis a consideration, but repeated serologic testing was negative.

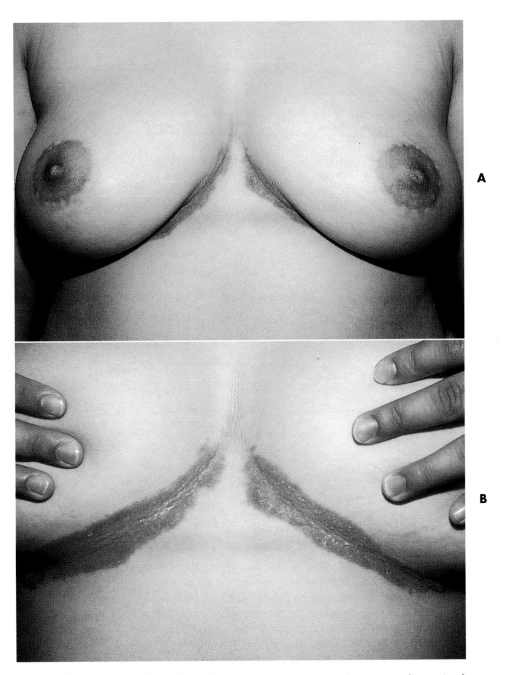

Figure 7-77 Inverse psoriasis. This Hispanic teenager developed psoriatic plaques in the inframammary folds 1 month before developing psoriasis of nearly her entire body surface.

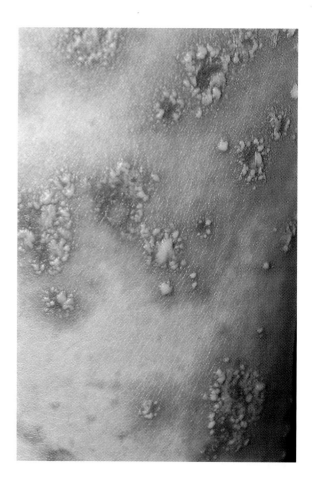

Figure 7-78   Pustular psoriasis in a 10-year old Filipino girl.

PYODERMA GANGRENOSUM

Clinical

Pyoderma gangrenosum (PG) may be separated into several clinical variants. The classic ulcerative type begins as a papule or pustule that breaks down to form an ulcer with an undermined, violaceous, jagged border. In pustular PG, painful, sterile pustules with a surrounding halo of erythema occur and may ulcerate (Figure 7-79). Fever, arthralgias, and the finding of inflammatory bowel disease are typical in pustular PG. In bullous PG, pseudovesicular lesions occur. In superficial granulomatous pyoderma, the lesions are more superficial, less aggressive, and more chronic (Figure 7-80). The edges are less violaceous. There is also a predilection for the trunk, and many patients do not have any associated diseases. Lesions of any form of PG may occur at sites of trauma (pathergy).

Associations

PG is classically associated with chronic inflammatory conditions such as ulcerative colitis, Crohn's disease, arthritis, chronic active hepatitis, and Takayasu's arteritis (as in Figure 7-79). An IgA paraprotein has been associated in approximately 10% of patients. Other diseases to exclude include lymphoma, deep funal infection, Wegener's granulomatosis, and the antiphospholipid syndrome.

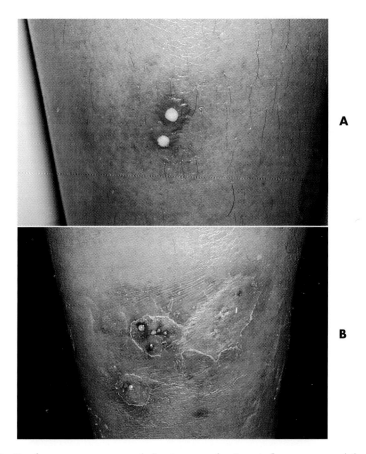

Figure 7-79   Pyoderma gangrenosum. **A,** Lesions may begin as inflammatory nodules or sterile pustules. **B,** Later, the area breaks down into multiple ulcerative, draining areas.

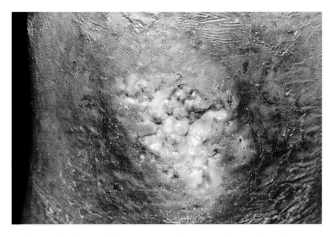

Figure 7-80   Superficial granulomatous pyoderma variant of pyoderma gangrenosum.

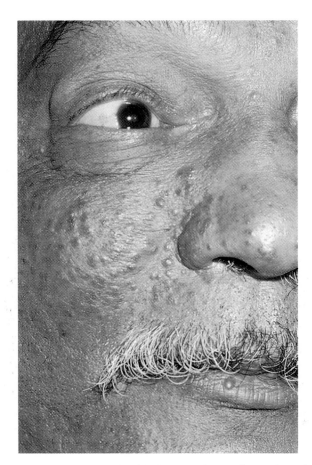

Figure 7-81   Papular rosacea in an adult black man. The condition cleared dramatically in a month on tetracycline 500 mg twice daily. Note the venous lake on the lower lip.

ROSACEA

Clinical

In whites, rosacea presents as papules and pustules of the central face. Rosacea is very uncommon in blacks, and when it does occur, it is often of the papular variety (Figure 7-81). Treatment with tetracycline 500 mg twice daily plus topical Metrogel or sodium sulfacetamide 10%/sulfur 5% is usually effective.

SCABIES

Scabies occurs with reasonable frequency in black children and adults. Any patient whose primary complaint is intense itching should have his or her hands and feet examined for the classic burrows of scabies (Figure 7-82). The penis and/or scrotum are often affected by erythematous nodules (Figure 7-83). Mineral oil examination showing the organism is diagnostic (Figure 7-84).

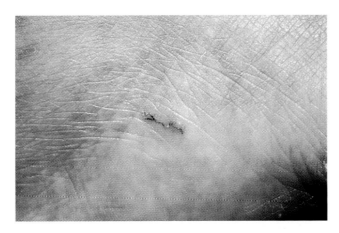

Figure 7-82 The classic burrow of scabies made more prominent by the ink test.

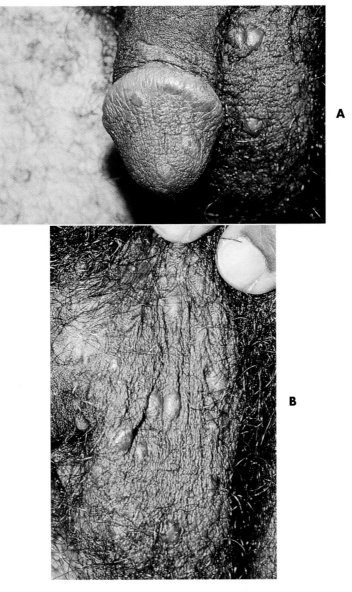

Figure 7-83 Nodular scabies of the penis **(A)** and scrotum **(B)**.

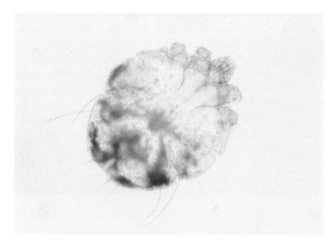

Figure 7-84   The scabies organism as seen on mineral oil examination.

SEBORRHEIC DERMATITIS

Etiology

Seborrheic dermatitis is a common inflammatory and scaly condition of the scalp, face, and ears of both blacks and whites. Various theories have been advanced as to the cause of seborrheic dermatitis. A favorite is that the lipophilic ("oil-loving") yeast Pityrosporum causes irritation of the skin. Infrequent shampooing makes the problem worse because it allows the organism to "overgrow." Although not supported by all studies, this theory is supported by the fact that "medicated" shampoos that are effective have antifungal activity, and the most effective shampoo, ketoconazole, has the most anti-Pityrosporum activity. This theory also explains why black patients have a tendency to develop seborrheic dermatitis (because they tend to shampoo less frequently than people of other races).

Clinical

Erythema and scale may affect the scalp, the skin about the ears, the nasolabial folds, the glabella, and elsewhere on the face (Figure 7-85). Annular forms may occur, and at times these changes blend into tinea versicolor on the neck and upper trunk (Figure 7-86). In blacks, postinflammatory hypopigmentation may occur on the face. Itching of the scalp is another common complaint.

Treatment

This condition is more easily treated in nonblacks because they can reasonably be asked to shampoo daily or every other day. Black individuals, however, because of culture and hairstyle, can only be reasonably asked to shampoo once or at most twice a

Seborrheic dermatitis is more easily treated in nonblacks because they can reasonably be asked to shampoo daily or every other day. Black individuals, however, because of culture and hairstyle, can only be reasonably asked to shampoo once or at most twice a week.

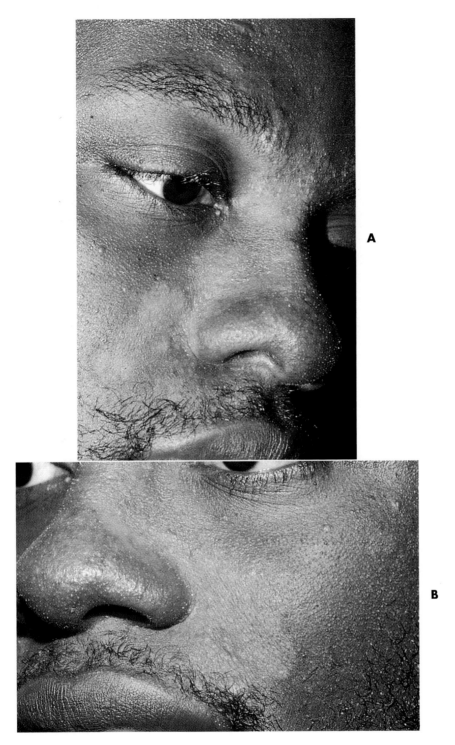

Figure 7-85   Seborrheic dermatitis.

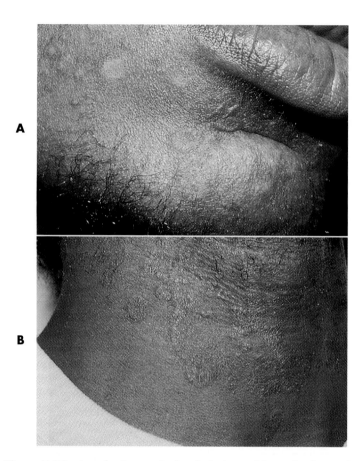

Figure 7-86   Annular forms of seborrheic dermatitis on the face and neck.

week. Medicated shampoos (e.g., ketoconazole 2%) should be recommended, and the patient should be instructed to let the shampoo sit on the scalp (contact with the hair is not necessary) for approximately 15 to 20 minutes. For those with significant itching or inflammation, a topical steroid should be added. A steroid ointment applied after shampooing is usually best and is appropriate for any type of hair—processed or hot-combed. It may also substitute for hair oils. Men with short hair or a shaved head may be reasonably asked to shampoo daily or every other day.

If seborrheic dermatitis is present on the face, the patient should be encouraged to lather the face as well as the scalp with the medicated shampoo. Later, either hydrocortisone 1% or ketoconazole creams may be applied.

SEBORRHEIC KERATOSIS

Seborrheic keratosis may occasionally be found. This growth is usually brown (Figure 7-87), but rarely it may be white (Figure 7-88).

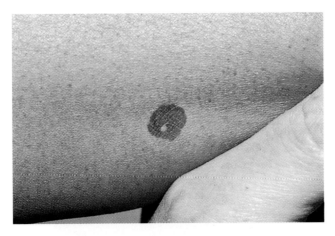

Figure 7-87   Seborrheic keratosis.

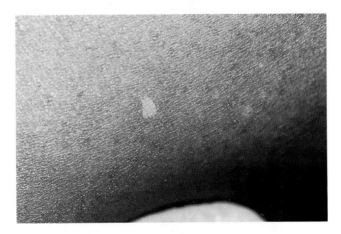

Figure 7-88   White seborrheic keratosis.

SEXUALLY TRANSMITTED DISEASES

The differential diagnosis of a penile ulcer has classically been comprised primarily of syphilis, chancroid, and granuloma inguinale. The ulcers of chancroid (Figure 7-89) tend to be painful and foul smelling. The organism involved is *Haemophilus ducreyi*, which has a "school of fish" appearance on smear. The ulcers of granuloma inguinale tend to be beefy yet asymptomatic, with exuberant granulation tissue (Figures 7-90 and 7-91). The organism involved is *Calymmatobacterium granulomatis*. The genital lesion of lymphogranuloma venereum is typically a small erosion that goes unnoticed until 1 to 2 weeks later, when firm lymphadenopathy develops (Figure 7-92). The classic "groove" sign is created by enlarged inguinal and femoral nodes separated by Poupart's ligament.

Secondary syphilis is similar in blacks and whites, with the exception that both a papular and an annular form are more common in the secondary syphilis of blacks.

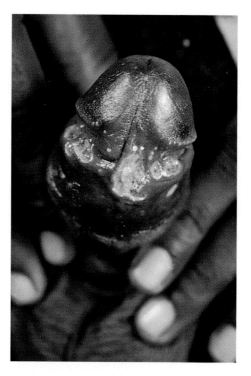

Figure 7-89   The differential diagnosis of a penile ulcer includes syphilis, chancroid, and granuloma inguinale. The diagnosis here—chancroid.

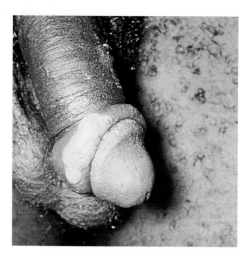

Figure 7-90   Granuloma inguinale.

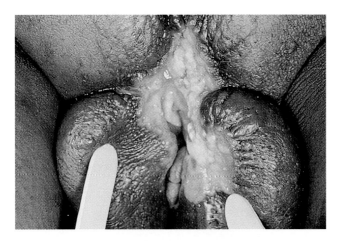

Figure 7-91   Marked labial edema in a patient with granuloma inguinale.

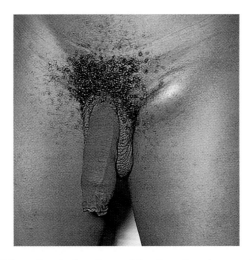

Figure 7-92   A large inguinal node resulting from lymphogranuloma venereum.

Syphilis has in the past been very common in the black population in both the United States and Africa. Its presentation is similar to that in whites, with divisions into primary, secondary, and tertiary syphilis. The classic ulcer of syphilis is usually shallow, firm, and painless. The organism is *Treponema pallidum* and can be viewed with darkfield examination of a smear. Secondary syphilis (Figures 7-93 and 7-94) is similar in blacks and whites, with the exception that both a papular and an annular form are more common in the secondary syphilis of blacks. The papular form may take on a variety of presentations, including disseminated or grouped, follicular or nonfollicular lesions. The annular presentation can be quite striking. Raised, annular, nickel- and dime-size lesions occur on the face (Figure 7-95), particularly about the mouth, nostrils, ears, and eyes. Secondary syphilis may also present as a moth-eaten alopecia (Figure 7-96) or condyloma lata (Figure 7-97). The skin lesions of tertiary (gummatous) syphilis are often polycyclic or serpiginous, with central clearing (Figure 7-98).

Condyloma accuminata caused by the human papilloma virus is a common sexually transmitted disease (Figure 7-99).

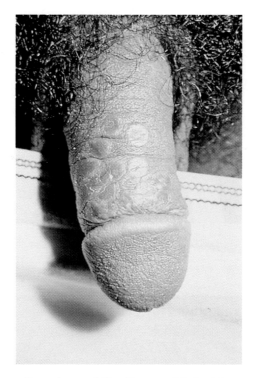

Figure 7-93   Secondary syphilis. (Courtesy Michael O. Murphy, MD.)

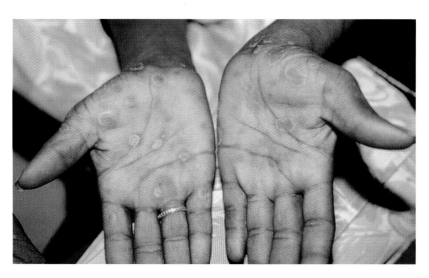

Figure 7-94   Involvement of the palms in secondary syphilis is classic. (Courtesy Steven Goldberg, MD.)

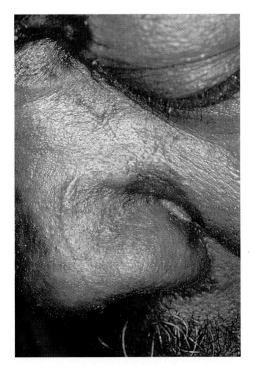

Figure 7-95 Annular forms of secondary syphilis on the face. (Courtesy Michael O. Murphy, MD.)

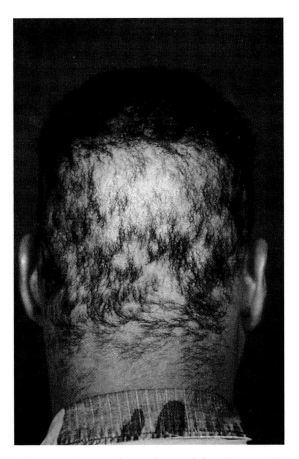

Figure 7-96 Moth-eaten alopecia of secondary syphilis. (Courtesy Stacy Smith, MD.)

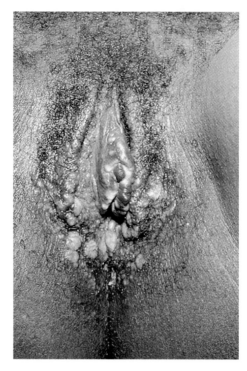

Figure 7-97   Condyloma lata of secondary syphilis. (Courtesy Michael O. Murphy, MD.)

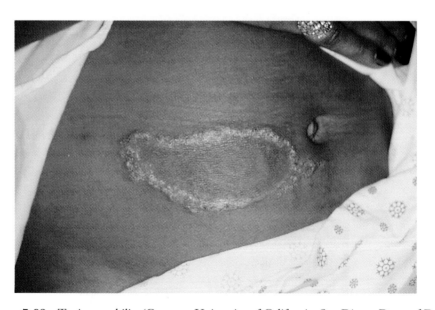

Figure 7-98   Tertiary syphilis. (Courtesy University of California, San Diego, Dept. of Dermatology.)

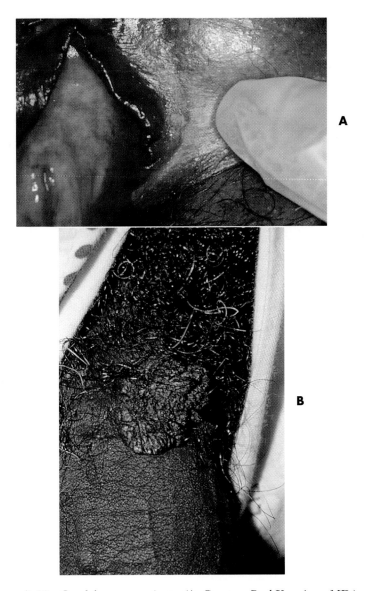

Figure 7-99   Condyloma accuminata. (**A,** Courtesy Paul Koonings, MD.)

STEATOCYSTOMA MULTIPLEX

Steatocystoma multiplex in blacks presents as multiple soft, cystic papulonodules of the chest, back, axilla, and arms (Figure 7-100). These papulonodules may range from 1 to 2 mm to 3 to 5 cm in size. The contents may be milky white or clear and oily. Rupture, inflammation, and scarring of individual cysts may occur and is called *steatocystoma multiplex suppurativa*. Excision of any cysts that have become large enough to be bothersome is the usual treatment (Figure 7-101).

TRICHOMYCOSIS AXILLARIS

Yellow, red, or black attachments on the hair representing bacterial colonization occur in trichomycosis axillaris (Figure 7-102). *Corynebacterium tenuis* is one of the bac-

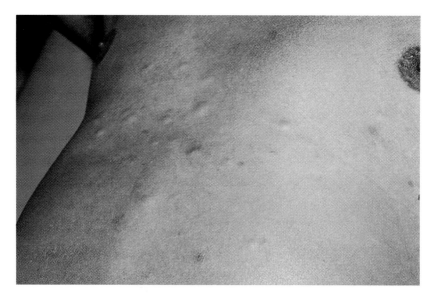

Figure 7-100   Multiple steatocystoma multiplex nodules of the chest are seen.

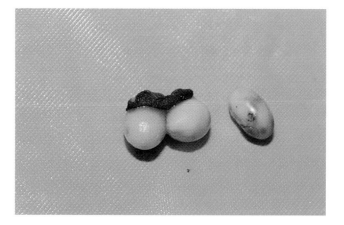

Figure 7-101   Multiple steatocystoma multiplex intact cysts after excision.

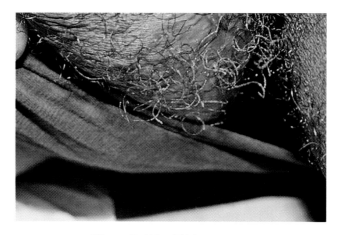

Figure 7-102   Trichomycosis.

teria that has been identified. Topical clindamycin twice daily or shaving are effective treatments.

URTICARIA AND DERMATOGRAPHISM

The typical pink color of urticaria is hidden in the darker-skinned patient. The lesions appear merely as itchy, nonscaly papules or plaques (Figure 7-103). It is the abrupt onset, the constantly changing character of the lesions, and the intense pruritus that help establish the diagnosis.

Patients with dermatographism usually present with the complaint of itching. The diagnostic feature is the development of linear wheals at the site of stroking (Figure 7-104). In the darker-skinned patient, the elevation and linearity are apparent, but the typical pink color is obscured. Diagnosis may be established by taking a tongue blade and stroking it several times across the back.

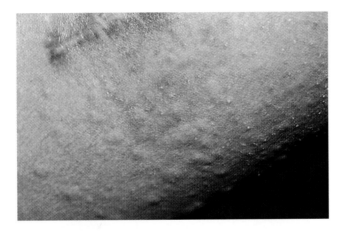

Figure 7-103   Urticaria. Note the raised wheals and the absence of the usual pink color.

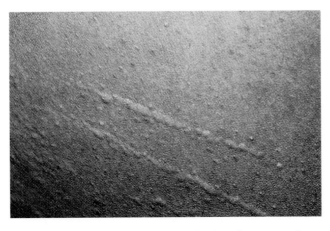

Figure 7-104   Dermatographism. A raised lesion developed minutes after scratching. Note the absence of visible erythema.

VENOUS LAKE

A dark blue, soft, compressible, vascular papule on the ears, lips, or face of an older person is characteristic of the venous lake. In the darker-skinned patient, the red/blue color is often obscured (Figure 7-105).

VERRUCA

Verruca (Figures 106 and 107) are less common in blacks compared with whites. For more information on verruca, see p. 152.

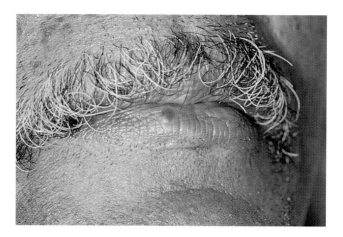

Figure 7-105   Venous lake.

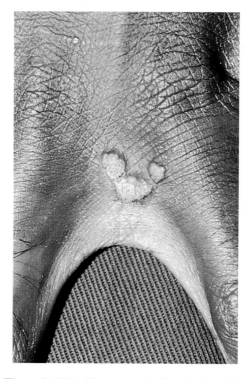

Figure 7-106   Verruca on the hand of an adult.

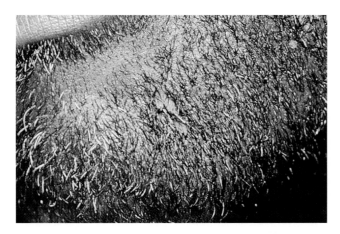

Figure 7-107   Filliform verruca on the face of an adult.

REFERENCES

1. Wilkins JW, Voorhees JJ: Prevalence of nodulocystic acne in white and negro males, *Arch Dermatol* 102:631-634, 1970.
2. Kaidbey KH, Kligman AM: A human model of coal tar acne, *Arch Dermatol* 109:212-215, 1974.
3. Halder RM et al: A clinicohistopathological study of acne vulgaris in black females, Poster presented at the 1997 AAD convention, San Francisco.
4. Bulengo-Ransby SM et al: Topical tretinoin (retinoic acid) therapy for hyperpigmented lesions caused by inflammation of the skin in black patients, *N Engl J Med* 328:1438-1443, 1993.
5. Pochi PE, Strauss JS: Sebaceous gland activity in black skin, *Dermatol Clin* 6:349-351, 1988.
6. Verhagen AR: Pomade acne in black skin (letter to the editor), *Arch Dermatol* 110:465, 1974.
7. Bulengo-Ransby SM et al: Topical tretinoin (retinoic acid) therapy for hyperpigmented lesions caused by inflammation of the skin in black patients, *N Engl J Med* 328:1438-1443, 1993.
8. Rietschel RL, Fowler Jr. JF, editors: *Fischer's contact dermatitis*, ed 4, Baltimore, 1995, Williams & Wilkins.
9. Fung MA et al: Confluent and reticulate papillomatosis: successful treatment with minocycline, *Arch Dermatol* 132:1400-1401, 1996.
10. George PM, Tunnessen WW: Childhood discoid lupus erythematosus, *Arch Dermatol* 129:613-617, 1993.
11. Goldstein E: Discoid lupus erythematosus: successful treatment with oral methotrexate, *Arch Dermatol* 130:938-939, 1994.
12. Knop J et al: Thalidomide in the treatment of sixty cases of chronic discoid lupus erythematosus, *Br J Dermatol* 108:461-466, 1983.
13. Shornick JK, Formica N, Parke AL: Isotretinoin for refractory lupus erythematosus, *J Am Acad Dermatol* 24:49-52, 1991.
14. Provost TT, Watson R, Simmons-O'Brien E: Significance of the anti-Ro(SS-A) antibody in evaluation of patients with cutaneous manifestations of a connective tissue disease, *J Am Acad Dermatol* 35:147-169, 1996.
15. Zackheim HS et al: Mycosis fungoides presenting as areas of hypopigmentation, *J Am Acad Dermatol* 6:340-345, 1982.
16. Whitmore SE, Simmons-O'Brien, Rotter FS: Hypopigmented mycosis fungoides, *Arch Dermatol* 130:476-480, 1994.
17. Breathnach SM, McKee PH, Smith NP: Hypopigmented mycosis fungoides: report of five cases with ultrastructural observations, *Br J Dermatol* 106:643-649, 1982.

18. Owen WR, Wood C: Disseminate and recurrent infundibulofolliculitis, *Arch Dermatol* 115:174-175, 1979.
19. Callot V et al: Drug-induced pseudolymphoma and hypersensitivity syndrome, *Arch Dermatol* 132:1315-1321, 1996.
20. Kromann NP, Bvilhelmsen R, Stahl D: The dapsone syndrome, *Arch Dermatol* 118:531-532, 1982.
21. Potter T et al: Dilantin hypersensitivity syndrome imitating staphylococcal toxic shock, *Arch Dermatol* 130:856-858, 1994.
22. Shear NH, Speilberg SP: Anticonvulsant hypersensitivity syndrome, *J Clin Invest* 82:1826-1832, 1988.
23. Troost RJ et al: Exfoliative dermatitis due to immunologically confirmed carbamazapine hypersensitivity, *Ped Dermatol* 13:316-320, 1996.
24. Handfield-Jones SE et al: The anticonvulsant hypersensitivity syndrome, *Br J Dermatol* 129:175-177, 1993.
25. Kopf AW et al: Prevalence of nevocytic nevi on lateral and medial aspects of arms, *J Dermatol Surg Oncol* 4:153-158, 1978.
26. Jacyk WK: Pityriasis rosea in Nigerians, *Int J Dermatol* 19:397-399, 1980.
27. Ahmed MA: Pityriasis rosea in the Sudan, *Int J Dermatol* 19:184-185, 1986.
28. Grimalt R et al: Pityriasis rotunda: report of a familial occurrence and review of the literature, *J Am Acad Dermatol* 31:866-871, 1994.
29. Obasi OE: Psoriasis vulgaris in the Guinea Savanah region of Nigeria, *Int J Dermatol* 25:181-183, 1986.

Common Pediatric Skin Diseases as They Appear in Dark Skin

Gary M. White

T his chapter presents a series of pictures and a brief discussion of common diseases as they appear in the dark-skinned child. When possible, special features prominent in black skin are noted.

Congenital/Neonatal Dermatology

CAFÉ AU LAIT SPOTS

A café au lait spot (CALS) is a congenital, fixed, brown macule or patch. It is uniform in color, with sharp borders and normal skin markings. It may be very small (Figure 8-1) or very large (Figure 8-2). Black children more commonly have CALSs than do white children. In one study of 4641 newborns, the incidence of at least one CALS was 0.3% for whites, 3.2% for Hispanics, and 12% for blacks.[1] No white newborn had more than one. In contrast, 4.4% of black newborns had at least two and 1.8% had at least three. Of note, a significant localization on the buttocks was noted, as was a lack of spots on the scalp.

Histologically, CALSs show macromelanosomes within the melanocyte and the keratinocyte. In one study, the size of the melanocyte was not changed.

Seven giant CALSs were also noted in the study by Alper and Holmes.[1] Six of the seven affected infants were black, and one was of mixed white and black descent. The incidence in the black infants was 1.2%. The buttocks and posterior leg were most commonly involved. Some stopped at the midline, but no true dermatome was involved in any of the cases. None of the infants at follow-up examinations years later showed any evidence of a neurocutaneous syndrome. Thus the giant CALS appears to be a benign entity. A biopsy of one lesion showed changes consistent with a CALS (i.e., increased size and activity of basal melanocytes).

NEVUS DEPIGMENTOSUS

A nevus depigmentosus is a congenital, stable, hypopigmented (but not depigmented) patch. It may be located randomly (Figure 8-3, *A*), segmentally (Figure 8-3, *B*),

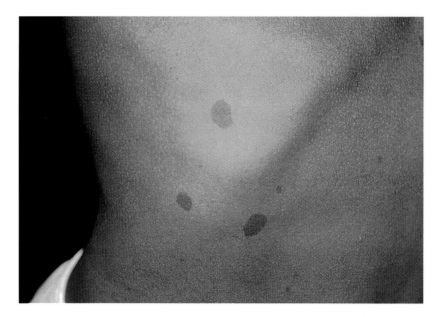

Figure 8-1   Café au lait spots. (Courtesy Paul J. Honig, MD.)

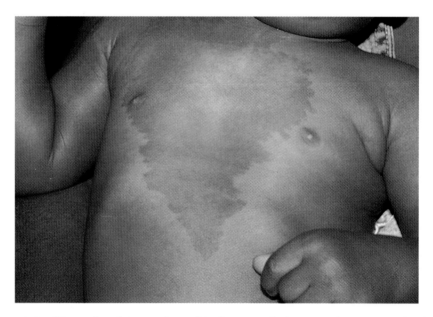

Figure 8-2   Giant café au lait spot. Giant CALSs seem to be benign and unassociated with any internal problems.

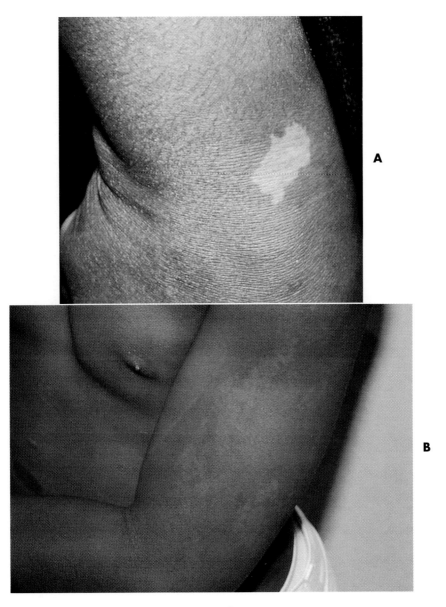

Figure 8-3   Nevus depigmentosus.

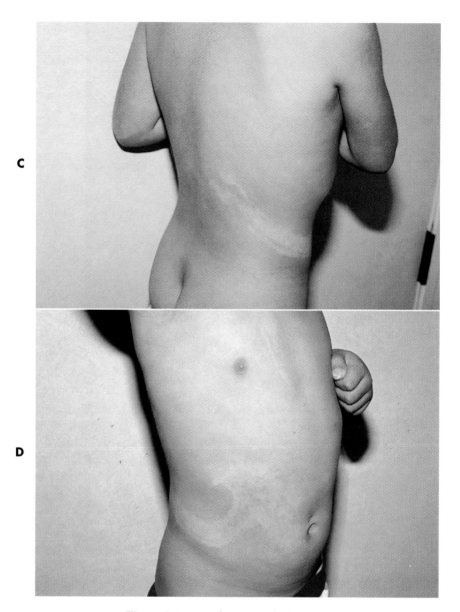

Figure 8-3, cont'd   Nevus depigmentosus.

linearly (Figure 8-3, *C*), or in a whorled pattern following Blaschko's lines* (Figure 8-3, *D*). When following Blaschko's lines, congenital systemic abnormalities may be associated. The Hispanic boy in Figure 8-3, *C* and *D* also had an artificial left eye.

MONGOLIAN SPOTS

For a discussion of mongolian spots, see p. 235.

---

*Alfred Blaschko, a private practitioner of dermatology in Berlin, transposed the linear pattern of more than 140 patients' skin lesions onto dolls and statues. His composite diagram has since been referred to as Blaschko's lines, and many skin diseases are distributed according to his pattern. Blaschko's lines are thought to result from the dorsoventral outgrowth of two different cell populations during early embryogenesis.

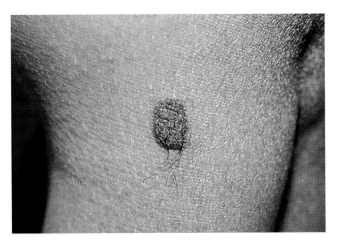

Figure 8-4   Congenital nevus.

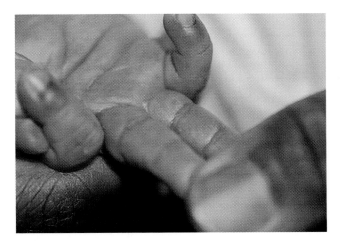

Figure 8-5   Transient neonatal pustular melanosis. Small pustules on the fingers are shown here. Infantile acropustulosis should be excluded.

CONGENITAL NEVI

Although black patients are more likely to have congenital nevi (Figure 8-4) than white patients (2% to 3% versus 1%), they are much less likely to develop melanoma in these lesions. Thus routine removal of such lesions is probably not necessary. Some physicians have modified this general approach by recommending the removal of congenital nevi in acral locations, especially the soles. Their rationale is that when melanoma does occur in blacks, it commonly presents in those locations.

TRANSIENT NEONATAL PUSTULAR MELANOSIS

Transient neonatal pustular melanosis preferentially occurs in the black infant, with an incidence of approximately 4% to 5%. It is a transient vesicopustular eruption (Figure 8-5) that is usually present at birth and ruptures within 24 to 48 hours, leaving a hyperpigmented macule. The face is a common site of involvement, but nearly any area may be affected. A smear of the lesion reveals both eosinophils and neutrophils, al-

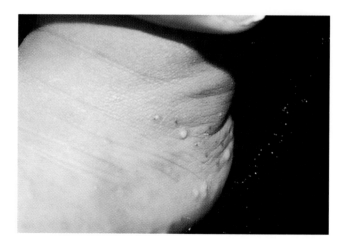

Figure 8-6 Multiple pustules of infantile acropustulosis on the heel of a black infant.

though this procedure is usually not needed to make the diagnosis. No treatment is required for this self-limiting disease.

INFANTILE ACROPUSTULOSIS

Clinical

Infantile acropustulosis is an uncommon pustular eruption that occurs primarily in infancy.[2] Its relationship to scabies remains unclear. Some cases may represent a hypersensitivity to the mite, whereas others seem unrelated. Confusing the clinical situation is the fact that many patients are treated empirically with antiscabetic preparations. Thus a hypersensitivity reaction to persistent mite antigens is difficult to completely exclude in some patients. Peripheral eosinophilia is present in many cases.

Clinically, the infant or young child presents with recurrent crops of 1- to 3-mm pruritic pustules on the distal extremities, especially the palms and soles (Figure 8-6). Less commonly, the trunk and even the face may be affected. The lesions last 1 to 2 weeks, and recurrences every several weeks to a month are common. Bacterial culture and scabies preparations should be done and are negative by definition.

Treatment

A potent topical steroid (e.g., betamethasone dipropionate, applied at bedtime for 1 to 2 days) is usually sufficient. Dapsone (e.g., 2 mg/kg/day) is effective treatment for infantile acropustulosis, but potential side effects make it less desirable. In particular, blacks with a deficiency of glucose-6-phosphate dehydrogenase should avoid this medication.

INCONTINENTIA PIGMENTI

Clinical

Although incontinentia pigmenti is not more common in darker-skinned patients, the pattern of hyperpigmentation can be quite dramatic in this population. Female infants are affected first by erythematous, vesicular, linear lesions and then by hyperkeratotic linear plaques that finally resolve, leaving linear and reticulated hyperpigmentation (Figure 8-7). The initial vesiculobullous phase is usually present at birth or develops in the first 2 weeks of life; the verrucous second stage is present from the sec-

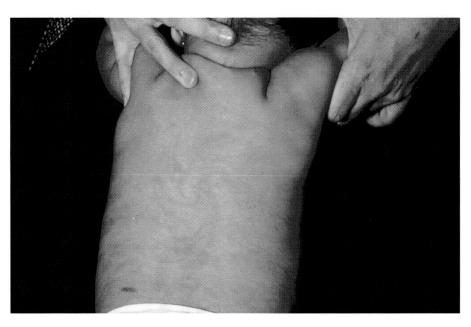

Figure 8-7   Pigmentary changes of incontinentia pigmenti. (Courtesy James Steger, MD.)

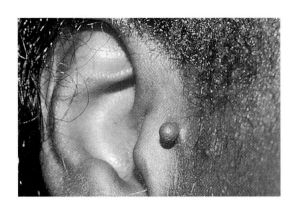

Figure 8-8   Accessory tragus.

ond to the sixth weeks, and the third pigmentary stage is most apparent from 12 to 26 weeks. Multisystem defects also occur, with preference for the musculoskeletal system, brain, eyes, hair, and teeth. This X-linked dominant disease only rarely affects males.

Treatment

No treatment is indicated for the skin changes. The noncutaneous changes are of greatest concern, and the patient should be evaluated and followed for those changes. Genetic counseling should also be provided.

ACCESSORY TRAGUS

Accessory tragi appear as congenital, firm nodules or pedunculated lesions in the preauricular area (Figure 8-8). They may occasionally be bilateral, are familial, and may occur in association with other facial abnormalities.

Pediatric Dermatology ————————————————

ACANTHOSIS NIGRICANS

Clinical

A brown, velvety thickening of the skin on the neck (Figure 8-9), axilla (Figure 8-10), elbows, and dorsa of the hands occurs in acanthosis nigricans.[3] This condition is extremely common, with an incidence of 7.1% in one study of 1412 children.[4] When these children were studied by race, non-Hispanic white children had an incidence of less than 1%. In Hispanics, the prevalence was 5.5%, and in blacks it was 13.3%. The presence of acanthosis nigricans is also associated with hyperandrogenism, insulin resistance, and obesity.

A common underlying cause of acanthosis nigricans appears to be elevated insulin levels. Overt diabetes is often not present because the pancreas is able to compensate. In one study that compared children with acanthosis nigricans and obesity with similarly obese children without acanthosis nigricans, the obese children with acanthosis nigricans were found to have higher insulin levels, higher HbA1c, and higher triglyceride levels.[5] The insulin was somewhat higher after fasting but significantly higher 1

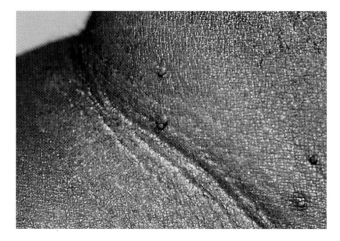

Figure 8-9   Acanthosis nigricans on the side of the neck. Several tags are seen as well.

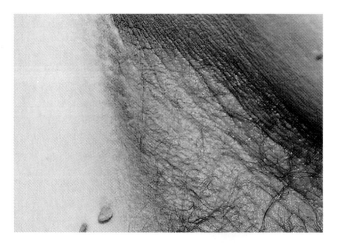

Figure 8-10   The typical velvety changes of acanthosis nigricans are seen in the axilla of this adult. Tags are common as well.

hour after a glucose challenge. The elevated HbA1c suggests that the elevated insulin levels do not fully compensate for the insulin resistance. The key point for clinical practice is to measure fasting insulin (and glucose) levels in children who have acanthosis nigricans, especially when it presents in unusual locations (Figure 8-11).

A common underlying cause of acanthosis nigricans appears to be elevated insulin levels.

Treatment

If a drug is causative, its use should be discontinued. Usually, however, one is faced with an obese child who seems otherwise healthy, but has acanthosis nigricans. Tretinoin has been used with some patients, although irritation may occur. Consider beginning with Retin-A 0.05% cream at bedtime applied to a test site. The greater concern is long term for two reasons: (1) diabetes may develop and (2) insulin resistance has been found to be an independent risk factor for coronary heart disease in adults. Weight loss, exercise, and periodic monitoring for the development of diabetes is recommended. Unfortunately, weight loss and maintenance of a normal weight seem to be empirically unsuccessful in this patient population.

ATOPIC DERMATITIS

Most clinicians can recognize a patient with atopic dermatitis, but agreeing on distinct diagnostic criteria is difficult. Regardless of the patient's race, the following factors are considered important.

1. An "eczematous" rash in an appropriate distribution. An eczematous lesion is characterized by redness, scale, and a somewhat ill-defined border. The distribution for infants may be diffuse, including the cheeks and the extensor surface of the extremities; for young children, it tends to be flexural (Figure 8-12). For adolescents and adults, flexural lesions, hand and periorbital dermatitis (Figure 8-13), and periauricular eczema are common. For all, varying amounts of excoriation and lichenification occur (Figure 8-14).
2. A personal or family history of asthma and/or seasonal rhinoconjunctivitis.
3. Itching.
4. A chronic course.

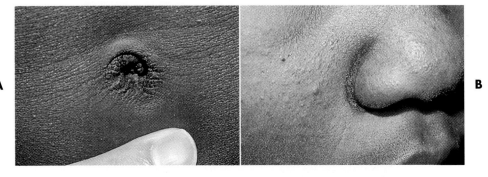

A   **B**

Figure 8-11   When acanthosis nigricans occurs in an unusual location in a child, the fasting insulin level is often elevated, as was true in both of these patients.

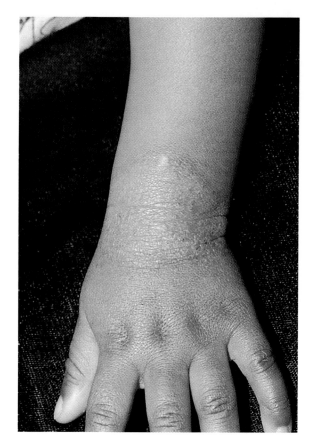

Figure 8-12 Flexural atopic dermatitis in an infant.

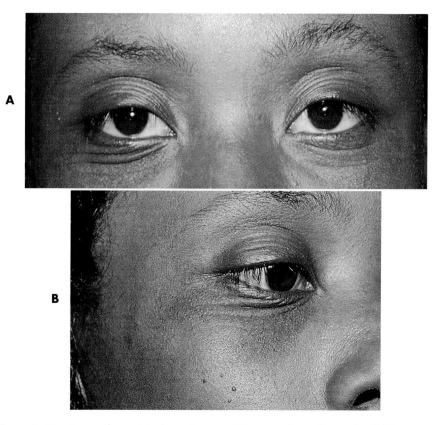

Figure 8-13 Atopic dermatitis about the eyes. Edema, scale, and excessive folding are seen.

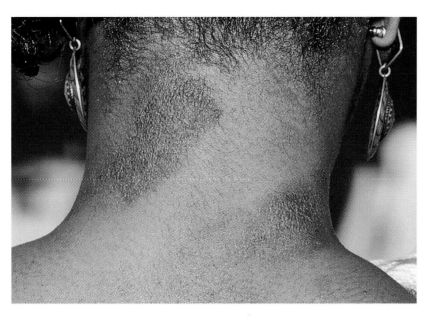

Figure 8-14   Lichen simplex chronicus in atopic dermatitis. The neck is a common site. Note the thickened skin and the accentuated skin folds.

Commonly associated (minor) features include dry skin, hyperlinear palms, Dennie's or Morgan's folds (multiple creases below the eyes), increased IgE reactivity, and increased tendency to infection by *Staphylococcus* and herpes simplex virus.

Additional features in blacks are erythema that may be difficult or impossible to see, follicular prominence, and tendency toward hyperpigmentation and hypopigmentation.

Atopic dermatitis is one of the most common skin conditions for which black children see the doctor. Some ethnic subpopulations may actually be more commonly affected. For example, London-born black children of Caribbean descent were found to have atopic dermatitis in 16.3% of cases, compared with 8.7% of white children.[6]

Follicular prominance is a characteristic feature of atopic dermatitis in black patients (Figure 8-15). Indeed, some children may present with innumerable, tiny (1 mm), follicular papules spread over the trunk and extremities in the absence of the classic red, scaly lesions.

Follicular prominance is a characteristic feature of atopic dermatitis in black patients.

Postinflammatory hypopigmentation is common in infants (Figure 8-16). The child's parents must be reassured that repigmentation will result. However, in areas of long-standing eczema and scratching, a patchy area of complete depigmentation may occur that will not repigment (Figure 8-17). As a general rule, areas that are hypopigmented will repigment, but areas of complete depigmentation will not. A linear, hypopigmented line may occur across the bridge of the nose if the child too often engages

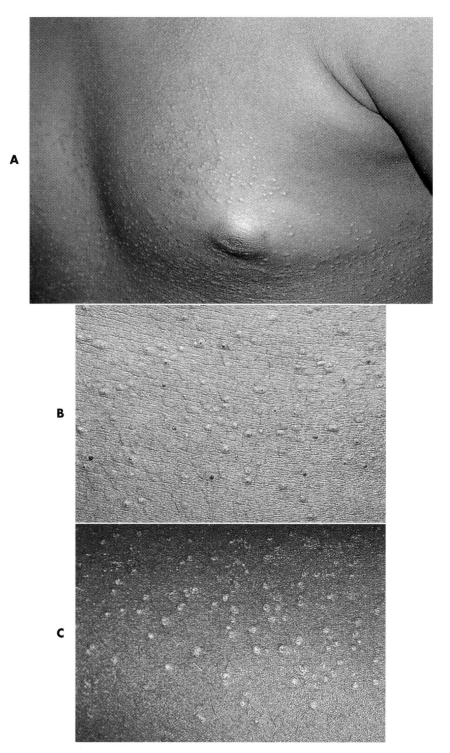

Figure 8-15   Follicular atopic dermatitis.

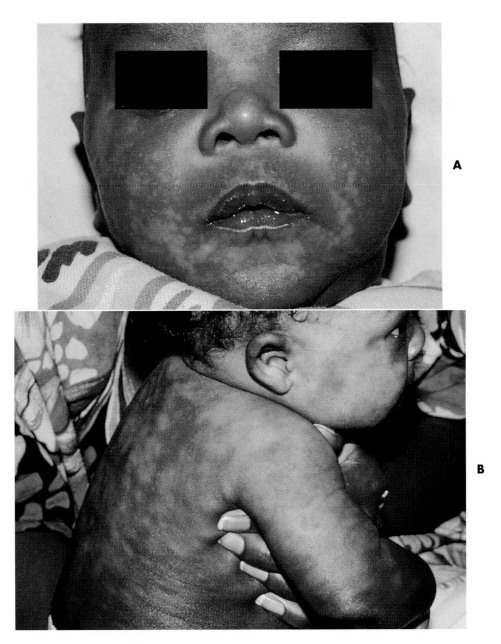

Figure 8-16   Postinflammatory hypopigmentation in an infant with atopic dermatitis.

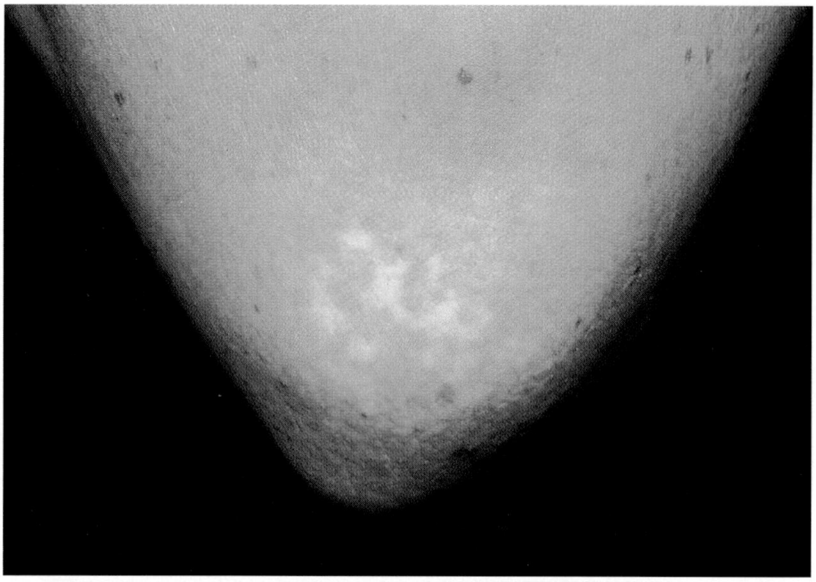

Figure 8-17   Complete loss of pigment in an area of long-standing atopic dermatitis.

in the allergic salute (Figure 8-18). Postinflammatory hyperpigmentation occurs as well, and some believe lichenification is more common in black patients. Unfortunately, atopic dermatitis may persist into the teenage or adult years (Figures 8-19 to 8-24).

Management

The clinical management of atopic dermatitis in the dark-skinned patient varies only slightly from that of other races. Specifically, a child's parents need to be reassured that pigmentation should normalize if the eczema is suppressed (except for completely depigmented areas [Figure 8-17]). Also, one must be careful not to cause hypopigmentation by using very strong topical corticosteroids (see p. 273). The following discussion of the treatment of atopic dermatitis is applicable to all races.

A child's parents need to be reassured that pigmentation should normalize if the eczema is suppressed.

The cornerstones of treatment for the patient with atopic dermatitis are (1) bathing habits, emolliation, and the application of topical steroids; (2) avoidance of trigger factors; and (3) not scratching. The primary activities of the doctor are (1) patient education and support, (2) management of flares, and (3) monitoring for and treating any superinfection.

Bathing habits and emollients

The patient with atopic dermatitis does not seem to make enough oils for the surface of his or her skin. Thus the skin dries out easily, and this is hastened by excessive bathing, water contact, and harsh soaps. Daily bathing is recommended, but baths or showers longer than 5 minutes should be avoided, and the water should not be hot. A mild (e.g., nondeodorant, nongreen) soap or cleanser should be used. An emollient should be applied to the skin within minutes of the bath or shower to "lock in" the

Text continued on p. 138

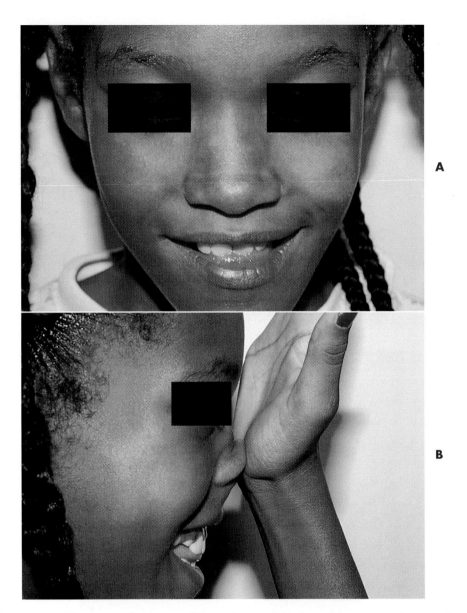

Figure 8-18 Transverse nasal groove. A hypopigmented, horizontal groove or stripe extending transversely across the nose may occur in a black child with atopic dermatitis **(A)** and allergic rhinitis. If watched carefully, the child will soon perform the allergic salute **(B).** This crease lies over the border between the alar and triangular nasal cartilages.

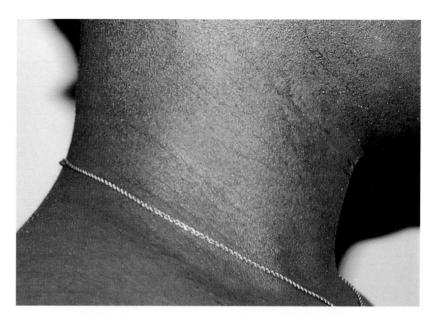

Figure 8-19 The "dirty neck" look of atopic dermatitis.

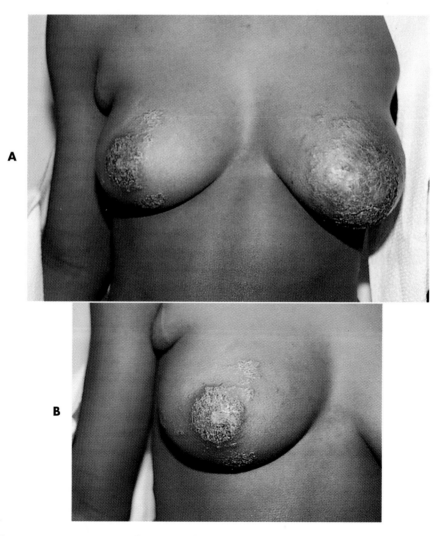

Figure 8-20 Eczematous changes of the nipples are not uncommon in atopic dermatitis as shown in this 14-year-old girl.

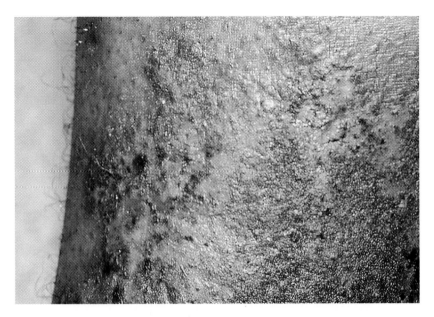

Figure 8-21   A lichenified plaque of lichen simplex chronicus on the shin of an adult.

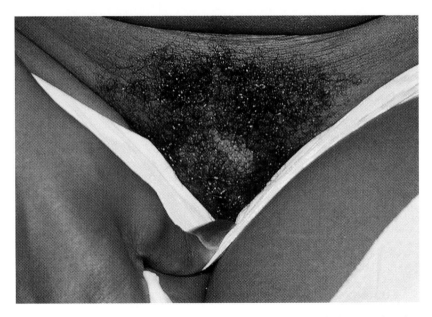

Figure 8-22   A lichenified plaque on the vulva identified as vulvar lichen simplex chronicus. The patient rubbed nightly.

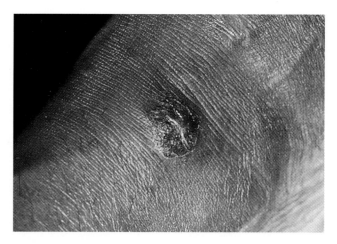

Figure 8-23   Prurigo nodule.

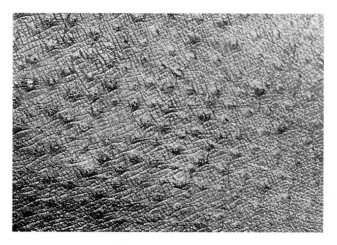

Figure 8-24   Follicular lichenification. An adult with atopic dermatitis who rubbed constantly developed lichenification with a follicular prominence.

moisture. The selection of the emollient should be individualized. Creams or ointments are best if tolerated. Lotions tend to have too much water and are best avoided, except in the mildest of cases.

Topical steroids

Emollients alone may be applied if the skin is just dry. However, when eczematous areas exist, a topical steroid is needed. The patient should be instructed to apply a low- to medium-potency steroid ointment to the eczematous areas and an emolliating cream or ointment to the rest of the skin. As a general rule, infants and those with mild disease may be improved sufficiently with hydrocortisone 1% to 2.5%. Children may be started on a class VI steroid. Adults may be initially given a class III or IV steroid. These are only starting points of treatment; if the patient is flaring, the physician usually has to go up a "notch" (class) on the steroid. Thus an infant flaring on hydrocortisone may need a class VI or V steroid. A young child flaring on a class VI steroid may need a class III. For the face, hydrocortisone is usually sufficient; rarely, a class VI or IV steroid is needed.

The steroid may be applied once more per day and the emollient 1 to 4 more times during the day during a flare, depending on the severity of the disease. It should be emphasized that the steroid should not be used as an emollient. The goal of therapy is routine maintenance with emollients only, with the use of steroids reserved for flares. The need to watch for steroid-induced hypopigmentation in the darker-skinned patient cannot be overemphasized.

Topical steroids combined with a course of oral antibiotics should be given to those patients with impetiginization or fissures and/or those not responding to therapy. In resistant cases, consider patient noncompliance or allergy to the topical steroid (switch to a different class for 2 to 3 weeks). Long pants and long-sleeved shirts may be helpful for children with significant involvement of the extremities. The clothing protects the skin from irritating dirt, carpet, and other allergens and decreases the tendency to scratch.

Avoiding trigger factors

Wool or other rough clothing may be irritating to the skin. The role of dust mite allergy is important for some patients, and testing by an allergist for this and other allergies is helpful. Various environmental control measures to reduce household exposure may be tried. For patients with prick test positivity to the dust mite, reduction of this allergen can be helpful. Patients may use a Goretex bedcover, wash their sheets weekly, spray benzyl-tannate to their bedroom and living-room carpets every 3 months, and use a high-filtration vacuum cleaner weekly. Irritation of the eyes by chlorine or cigarette smoke has also been reported. Various foods can exacerbate atopic dermatitis, especially in children. The most common food allergens are eggs, peanuts, milk, fish, soy, and wheat. However, there is currently no reliable test to definitively establish such a cause and effect. A good history, radioallergosorbent test (RAST), and food challenge tests may be helpful. Referral to an allergist is often indicated, especially for treatment-resistant patients under 2 years of age. Undirected elimination diets should be avoided. Whether stress alone can cause a flare of atopic dermatitis is unclear. For some, sweating can cause pruritus, scratching, and thus more eczema. Most patients are worse during dry, cold winters, but some may experience exacerbations during the summer.

A good history, RAST testing, and food challenge tests may be helpful. Referral to an allergist is often indicated, especially for treatment-resistant patients under 2 years of age. A "flare" of AD may in reality represent superinfection with either S. aureus *or herpes simplex virus.*

Patient education

Educating the parent about the cause of atopic dermatitis, basic skin care, and what to do when a child flares is of vital importance. Both verbal instruction and written handouts are important. Creative ways of helping the child not scratch are often discussed (e.g., gloves sewn onto pajamas).

Superinfection

Every atopic patient flares. When a child does, a parent will call the doctor, seeking advice. It is important for every physician who cares for patients with atopic dermatitis to understand that a "flare" of atopic dermatitis may in reality represent superinfection with either *S. aureus* or herpes simplex virus. Thus it is usually necessary to see the patient. Appropriate therapy may then be instituted with either an antistaphylococcal antibiotic or an oral antiviral agent (e.g., acyclovir). If no superinfection has occurred, increasing the potency of the topical steroid for a week or so may be all that is

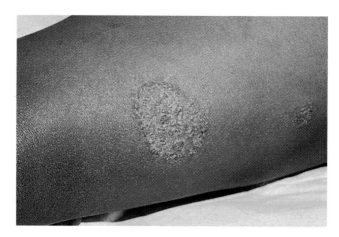

Figure 8-25   Nummular eczema in a child.

needed. Alternatively, an oral antistaphylococcal antibiotic may be given even in the absence of overt infection.

Sleep difficulties

One study found that children with atopic dermatitis who have sleep difficulties usually experience them during atopic dermatitis flares and may keep their parents up an average of 2 to 3 hours. Strategies rated by the parents as most successful at these times were putting creams on the child, using cotton clothes, keeping the room cool, putting very few blankets over the child, and cuddling the child. Bringing the child into the parents' bed seems to prolong the problem.

NUMMULAR ECZEMA

Nummular eczema is a specific variant of eczema and is seen in both children and adults. Coin-shaped (Figure 8-25) (nummular), red, eczematous areas are characteristic and are common on the arms and legs. The surface may be oozing and crusted or dry and scaly. Pruritis may be significant. Risk factors include excessive time in the bath (e.g., more than 10 minutes) or other situations involving prolonged water exposure (e.g., swimming).

Prolonged water exposure should be avoided. A medium- to high-potency topical steroid ointment should be applied after the bath or shower. Systemic steroids may be given if the lesions are widespread and/or resistant to topical treatment. Vaseline or a heavy cream applied to the skin immediately after the bath or shower helps prevent future outbreaks. Lotions should not be used.

BECKER'S NEVUS

An acquired, pigmented patch with hair on the trunk is characteristic of a Becker's nevus (Figure 8-26). Onset is usually in the preteen years. No treatment is effective. The lesion is usually of cosmetic concern only.

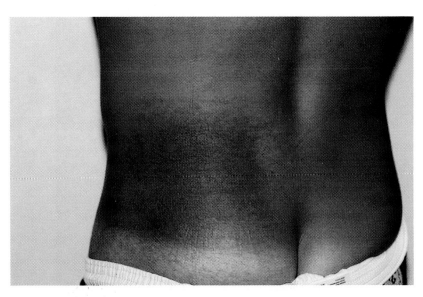

Figure 8-26   Becker's nevus. An acquired pigmented patch with hair is characteristic of a Becker's nevus and is shown here on the flank of a 10-year-old boy. No treatment is effective. The lesion is usually of cosmetic concern only.

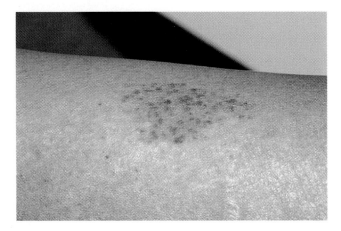

Figure 8-27   Nevus spilus. These speckled, lentiginous nevi may occasionally occur in black patients. No treatment is needed.

NEVUS SPILUS

The speckled, lentiginous nevi of nevus spilus may occasionally occur in black patients (Figure 8-27). The nevi are characterized by multiple, grouped, pigmented macules. The background may be the color of normal skin or slightly hyperpigmented.

ICTHYOSIS

Ichthyosis may affect those with darker skin. The most common form is ichthyosis vulgaris (Figure 8-28), which is inherited in an autosomal dominant fashion. Severe

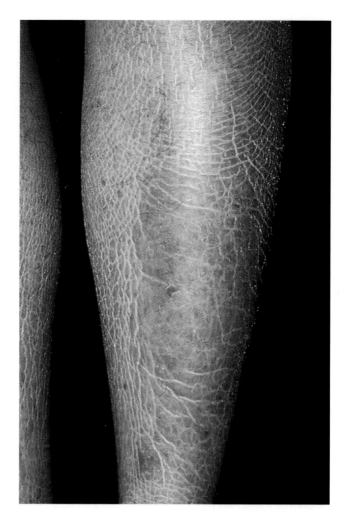

Figure 8-28   Icthyosis vulgaris.

xerosis and fine scaling with onset in the first few months of life is characteristic. In comparison with other forms of ichthyosis, the skin changes of ichthyosis vulgaris are mild. The disease is worse in the winter, is commonly seen on the legs, and may worsen with age. The scales of recessive X-linked ichthyosis (Figure 8-29) are larger, darker, and thicker compared with ichthyosis vulgaris. The flexures are usually spared. Males are affected, although carrier females may exhibit mild features as well as failure to go into labor spontaneously. The scales of lamellar ichthyosis are also larger than those of ichthyosis vulgaris. The patient often presents as a collodion baby at birth. Later, the skin becomes ichthyotic, with large platelike scales and variable erythroderma. Ectropion and palmoplantar keratoderma are frequently present. Inheritance is autosomal recessive.

IMPETIGO

A tiny pustule or vesicle forms initially and then rapidly spreads to form the typical honey-colored, crusted lesion. Lesions may be pustular, crusted (Figure 8-30),

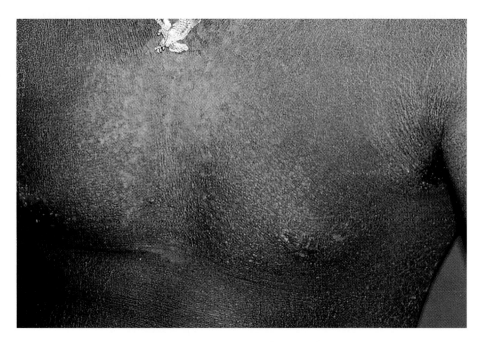

Figure 8-29   Recessive X-linked icthyosis.

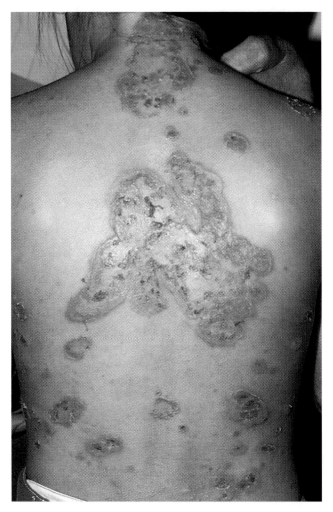

Figure 8-30   Widespread impetigo in a Filipino child.

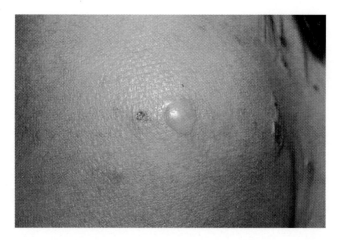

Figure 8-31   Bullous impetigo. A bullous lesion with a pus/fluid line.

bullous (Figure 8-31) or mixed. The erythema is often obscured in the darker-skinned patient. Pain, surrounding erythema, and constitutional symptoms are usually absent. Regional adenopathy is common. *S. aureus* or *Streptococcus pyogenes* are the usual pathogens, with *S. aureus* being more common. Chickenpox, insect bites, abrasions, lacerations, and burns commonly precede nonbullous impetigo. Atopic dermatitis patients are usually highly colonized with *S. aureus* and are at increased risk for impetigo.

Topical mupirocin applied three times a day for 7 days may be given for localized disease, although it probably should not be used around the mouth because it may be licked off. For widespread involvement, an oral antibiotic (e.g., cephalexin, dicloxacillin, or erythromycin, 30 to 50 mg/kg/day) is effective.

LICHEN NITIDUS

Clinical

In lichen nitidus, a curious disorder of unknown etiology, innumerable, monomorphous, 1-mm papules occur. Their surface is shiny, and many sites may be affected. The forearm, chest, abdomen, and penis are typical. Koebner's phenomenon (i.e., the occurrence of lesions at sites of skin trauma) is common. In the rare variant—lichen nitidus actinicus—the classic monomorphous papules occur only in sunexposed areas (Figure 8-32).

Histologic examination of a papule shows an infiltrate in one or two dermal papillae that consist of lymphocytes, histiocytes, and often granulomas. The overlying epidermis is atrophic, and the lateral rete are acanthotic and enclose the infiltrate ("ball and claw" configuration).

Treatment

Observation is appropriate, but if treatment is needed, a medium- to high-potency topical steroid may be given. Other treatments for widespread involvement have in-

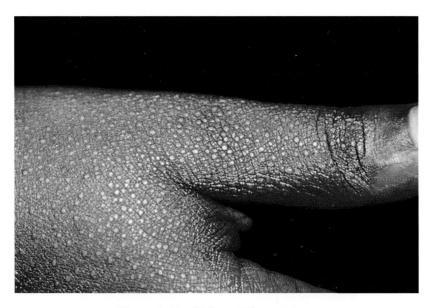

Figure 8-32 Lichen nitidus actinicus.

cluded PUVA,[8] etretinate, and acitretin.[9] For lichen nitidus actinicus, both a topical steroid and a sunscreen should be recommended.

LICHEN SCLEROSIS

Clinical

Lichen sclerosis is an unual condition characterized by atrophy of the skin. It tends to occur in young girls in the vulvar area. White, atrophic, crinkled, shiny areas with follicular plugging develop symmetrically about the vagina and rectum in an "hour-glass" appearance (Figure 8-33). Pruritus, burning pain, dyspareunia, dysuria, vaginal discharge, anal or genital bleeding, labial stenosis or fusion, constipation, erosion, contraction, and squamous cell carcinoma may occur. This can be a self-limiting condition in children.

Treatment

Clobetasol propionate (twice daily for 1 month, every day for 2 months, then twice weekly) is dramatically effective in most cases. The pruritus is greatly reduced within a week, but the clobetasol should be continued to reduce progressive scarring. Less potent topical corticosteroids have also been used. Wearing underwear helps prevent exposing the thighs to the effects of the steroid.

LICHEN STRIATUS

Clinical

Lichen striatus is a unique, inflammatory condition that usually presents in a child as lines, arcs, whorls, and swirls that follow Blaschko's lines. Its cause is unknown.

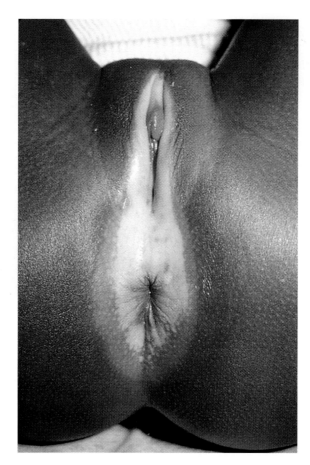

Figure 8-33 Lichen sclerosis of the groin in a young girl. (Courtesy Michael O. Murphy, MD.)

Clinically, one sees linear papules or red, scaly lesions that appear suddenly and follow Blaschko's lines (Figure 8-34). The child is often brought in as the lesion evolves. Several months may be needed before the lesions cease to progress. If the proximal nail fold is involved, nail dystrophy may occur (Figure 8-35). Itching is usually minimal to absent. In the darker-skinned patient, postinflammatory hypopigmentation is very common (Figure 8-36) and can be particularly distressing. In a series of 18 cases of lichen striatus, the mean age of onset was 3 years, the mean duration was 9.5 months, and hypochromic sequelae occurred in 50% of the cases.[10] Some have reported an association with atopy.

Histologic examination shows a nonspecific perivascular and lichenoid infiltrate. Epidermal changes of edema and exocytosis and/or parakeratosis are thought to represent secondary changes.

Treatment

No specific treatment is known to be effective. Lichen striatus usually involutes within a year. Topical steroids may be tried if needed, and intralesional steroids may be recommended in rare conditions to limited areas that persist.

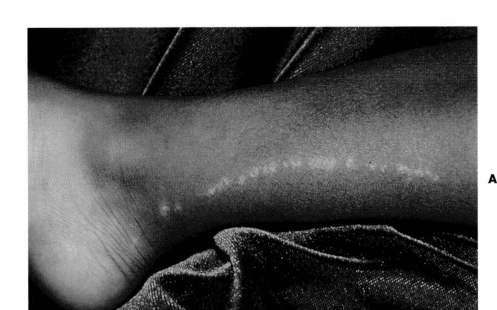

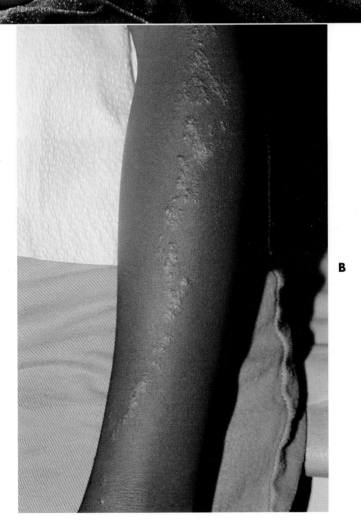

Figure 8-34   Lichen striatus.

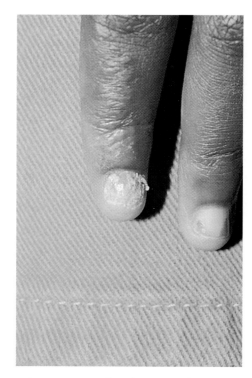

Figure 8-35   Lichen striatus may extend to the proximal nail fold, causing nail dystrophy.

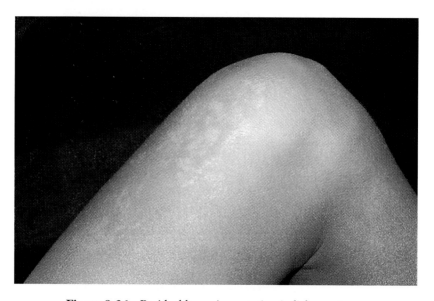

Figure 8-36   Residual hypopigmentation in lichen striatus.

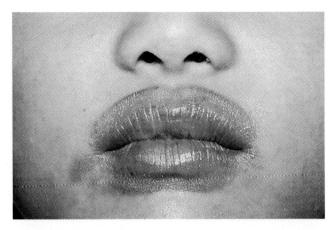

Figure 8-37   Only the skin accessible to the tongue is affected in lip-licking dermatitis.

LIP-LICKING DERMATITIS

Red, scaly, crusted, eczematous changes of the skin encircling the mouth in a child are characteristic of lip-licking dermatitis (Figure 8-37). Only that skin accessible to the tongue is affected. This represents an irritant contact dermatitis from the constant wetting and irritation by the saliva. The child should be encouraged to keep his tongue in his mouth. Vaseline may be applied to the affected area several times a day as a protectant.

PITYRIASIS ALBA

Clinical

Multiple hypopigmented, ill-defined areas that may be slightly scaly and that occur on the face and/or arms of a child are characteristic of pityriasis alba. The malar eminence of the cheeks is the most commonly affected spot (Figure 8-38). Though it occurs in all races, the primary manifestation—hypopigmentation—is more prominent in darker skin. Thus the presentation of pityriasis alba may never be seen in the very fair-skinned person, whereas its presentation in the darker-skinned patient is common. Pityriasis alba may be thought of as a variant of postinflammatory hypopigmentation after eczema. The history of a prior red, scaly, eczematous rash, however, may not be given by the patient. Patients are nearly always preadolescent, because increased sebum production in teenagers prevents the initial eczema.

The differential diagnosis should always include vitiligo; however, the patches of vitiligo are completely devoid of pigment and the edges are sharp. For hypopigmented areas on the upper arm, the back should also be examined to help exclude tinea versicolor. Occasionally, hypopigmented areas along the hairline or on the face that are interpreted as pityriasis alba are actually postinflammatory changes of either tinea versicolor or seborrheic dermatitis.

In the darker child, the center may occasionally take on a bluish hue because of pigmentary incontinence (melanin in the dermis). This appearance has been termed

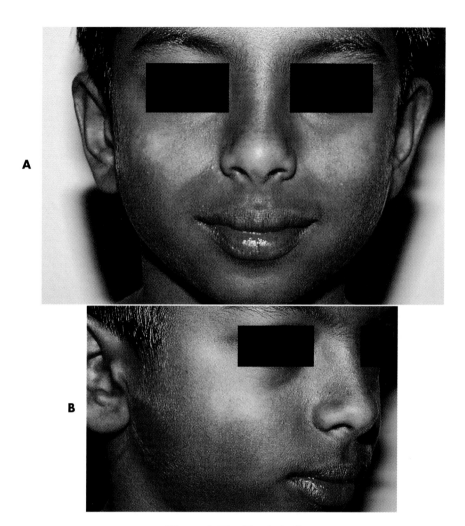

Figure 8-38 Pityriasis alba.

pigmenting pityriasis alba. It was initially thought to be a marker of dermatophyte infection, but we agree with Dhar, Kanwar, and Dawn[11] that it is not.

Treatment

The patient and his or her parents should be reassured that these changes are almost without exception reversible once the eczematous process is stopped. The return to normal pigment, however, occurs over several months, so patience is necessary. The less sun exposure the patient has, the better, because the normal skin will darken, making the pityriasis alba more obvious. Emollients and a mild topical steroid may be recommended. Hydrocortisone 1% cream is usually the only treatment that is needed initially, and it is followed several weeks later by an emolliating cream. Lotions are often not emolliating enough, and ointments are poorly tolerated.

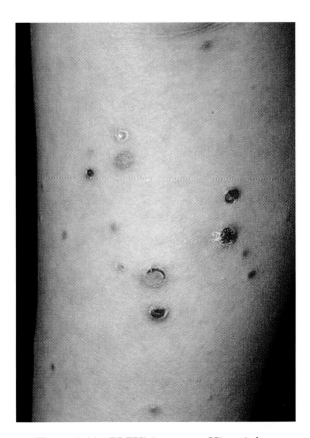

Figure 8-39   PLEVA in a young Hispanic boy.

PITYRIASIS LICHENOIDES ET VARIOLIFORMIS ACUTA

Clinical

Also known as *PLEVA*, pityriasis lichenoides et varioliformis acuta is common in people of all races, but can cause very distressing hypopigmentation in the darker-skinned patient. The patient initially develops many scattered, scaly papules and plaques on the extremities and trunk. These lesions often go on to develop a necrotic center followed by a crust (Figure 8-39). After healing, a hypopigmented macule is a common sequela. Fever and constitutional symptoms may accompany the outbreaks. The age of onset is from 1 year to old age, although it is most common in the first three decades. The disease may last from months to decades, with lesions often coming in crops. The condition must be differentiated from other papulosquamous conditions (e.g., psoriasis and pityriasis rosea). The presence of lesions in all stages of development and the necrotic central portion usually allows a diagnosis to be made without a biopsy.

Treatment

When significant hypopigmentation occurs, UVB may be indicated. If it fails and the patient is old enough, PUVA is an alternative. Otherwise, sunlight may help clear the lesions, and erythromycin for 2 to 4 months may also be prescribed. Tetracycline may also be tried with older children.

PITYRIASIS ROSEA (FIGURE 8-40)

See Chapter 7 for discussion.

PSORIASIS (FIGURE 8-41)

See Chapter 7 for discussion.

TINEA CAPITIS (FIGURE 8-42)

See p. 224 for discussion.

TRACTION ALOPECIA (FIGURE-8-43)

See p. 222 for discussion.

VERRUCA

Warts seem for some reason to be less common in black children (Figure 8-44). This is fortunate, because the most common treatment, cryotherapy, may cause temporary or permanent hypopigmentation. Salicylic acid, 17% to 23% applied daily; paring the lesion with a steel blade; or reducing it with a pumice stone every 2 to 4 days is appropriate therapy. Cryotherapy may be necessary, and its potential for hypopigmentation is less of a concern for those lesions on the palms or soles.

Warts seem for some reason to be less common in black children.

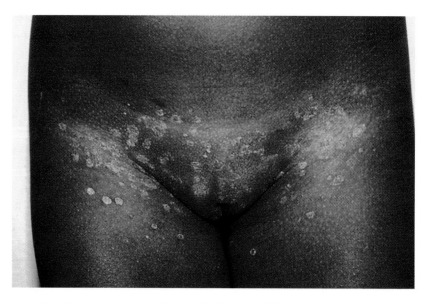

Figure 8-40   Pityriasis rosea in a 5-year-old black girl. Note the preference for the groin.

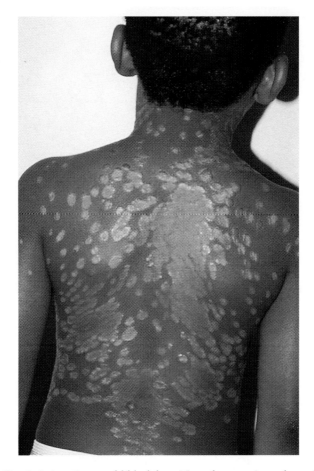

Figure 8-41 Psoriasis in a 5-year-old black boy. Note the prominent loss of pigmentation.

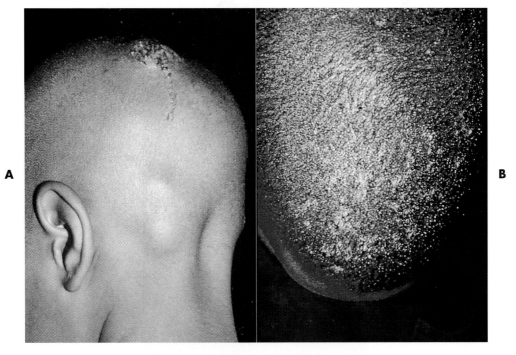

Figure 8-42 Tinea capitis. A fungal infection of the scalp may present as a boggy mass of tissue, or kerion, **(A)** or as scale alone, resembling seborrheic dermatitis **(B).** Note the swollen lymph node in **A.**

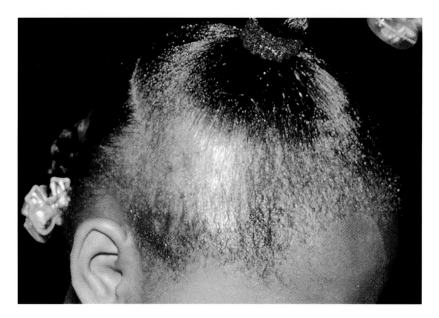

Figure 8-43   Traction alopecia.

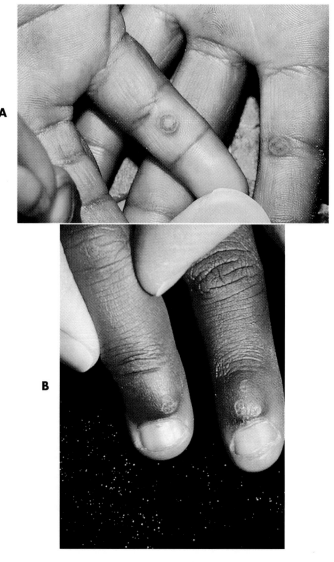

Figure 8-44   Verruca on the fingers of a child.

REFERENCES

1. Alper JC, Holmes LB: The incidence and significance of birthmarks in a cohort of 4641 newborns, *Pediatr Dermatol* 1:58-68, 1983.
2. Jarratt M, Ramsdell W: Infantile acropustulosis, *Arch Dermatol* 115:834-836, 1979.
3. Schwartz RA: Acanthosis nigricans, *J Am Acad Dermatol* 31:1-19, 1994.
4. Stuart CA, Pate CJ, Peters E: Prevalence of acanthosis nigricans in an unselected population, *Am J Med* 87:269-272, 1989.
5. Larry Eichenfield, MD, Chief of Pediatric Dermatology, Children's Hospital, San Diego, Calif, personal communication.
6. Williams HC et al: London-born black Caribbean children are at increased risk of atopic dermatitis, *J Am Acad Dermatol* 32:212-217, 1995.
7. Kanwar AJ, Surrinder K: Lichen nitidus actinicus, *Pediatr Dermatol* 8:94-95, 1991.
8. Randle HW, Sander HM: Treatment of generalized lichen nitidus with PUVA, *Int J Dermatol* 25:461-462, 1986.
9. Lucker GPH et al: Treatment of palmoplantar lichen nitidus with acitretin, *Br J Dermatol* 130:791-793, 1994.
10. Taieb A et al: Lichen striatus: a Blaschko linear acquired inflammatory skin eruption, *J Am Acad Dermatol* 25:637-642, 1991.
11. Dhar S, Kanwar AL, Dawn G: Pigmenting pityriasis alba, *Pediatr Dermatol* 12:197-198, 1995.

Chapter 9

Acne Keloidalis Nuchae

Gary M. White

Acne keloidalis nuchae is a chronic, progressive, keloidal scarring process of the nape in black men (Figure 9-1). Its cause is unknown. Treatment is difficult, and surgical intervention is often necessary.

EPIDEMIOLOGY

Acne keloidalis nuchae is predominantly a disease of young black men. Rarely, white or Asian men and even women[1] may be affected. Onset is usually after puberty, and most patients seek treatment in their 20s or 30s. A recent short haircut may precipitate the condition. The coexistence of pseudofolliculitis barbae has been noted in many patients, implying an underlying predisposition to both disorders, although there is no clinical or histologic evidence of recurring of superficial hairs into the skin in acne keloidalis nuchae. Acne vulgaris does not appear to be associated.

Acne keloidalis nuchae is predominantly a disease of young black men.

ETIOLOGY

Although the exact etiology is unknown, several steps in the development and progression of the disease are known. The initial histologic picture is that of follicular (or perifollicular) inflammation. Studies indicate that this inflammation begins somewhere between the insertion of the arrector pili muscle to just above the connection of the sebaceous duct. The follicular wall is weakened and ultimately ruptures. The release of the hair shaft into the dermis incites a foreign body response. Intense inflammation, transepidermal elimination of hair and debris, and scarring follow. Why the initial follicular inflammation occurs is unclear. Neither the changes of acne vulgaris (e.g., follicular hyperkeratinization with distention of the follicle) nor the changes of pseudofolliculitis barbae (e.g., inward curving of hairs causing penetration of the follicular wall or epidermis) are seen. Demodex has been demonstrated in acne keloidalis nuchae lesions, but its pathogenic involvement remains to be substantiated.

Infection can greatly contribute to the inflammation and scarring but is thought to be a secondary event. In one study, fasting serum testosterone levels were significantly elevated over controls, but the significance is unknown.[2] An autoimmune process has been suggested; however, supporting data are lacking.

156

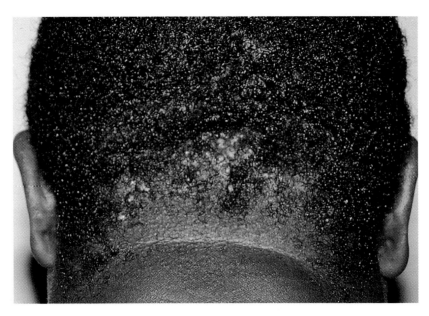

Figure 9-1   A papular rash on the nape of a black man's neck is almost always acne keloidalis nuchae.

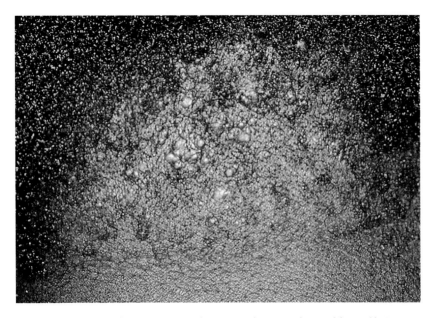

Figure 9-2   Close inspection shows papules, pustules, and loss of hair.

CLINICAL

A follicular, pustular eruption on the nape of the neck develops initially (Figure 9-2). Comedones are not seen. Later, firm follicular papules develop (Figure 9-3). Large keloids with sinus tracts, pus, and scarring alopecia may form. Inside the keloidal nodules are crypts of trapped hairs. Often, these groups of hairs eminate from one opening (tufted hairs or polytrichia) (Figure 9-4).

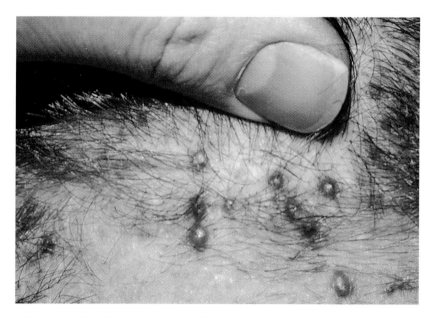

Figure 9-3 Acne keloidalis nuchae in a white man. Note the erythema here that is usually much less obvious in a darker-skinned patient.

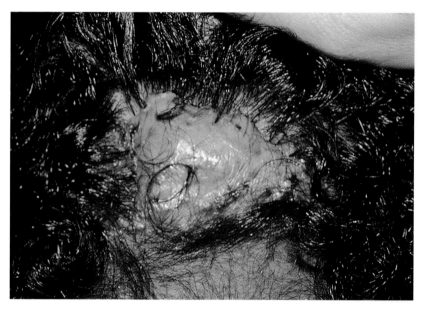

Figure 9-4 A large keloid has formed. Note the polytrichia seen in the upper portion of the keloid.

Small lesions may be asymptomatic. As the disease progresses, significant tenderness, itching, or burning may occur. Areas of alopecia and large keloids are cosmetically distressing. Drainage may stain clothes and cause an odor. One patient with a giant keloid was unable to sleep on his back and had an elaborate hairpiece to disguise his condition.[3]

Pustules, crusting, and drainage are usually manifestations of a secondary infectious component; occasionally, the inflammation is noninfectious, and cultures are sterile. When a bacteria is found, it is usually *S. aureus.* The occipital-posterior hairline is

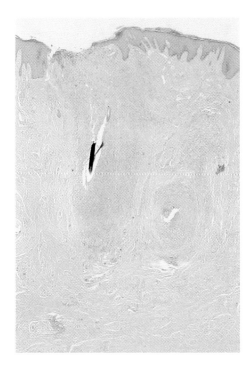

Figure 9-5   Perifollicular inflammation and follicular eruption. (Dermal fibrosis ×40.)

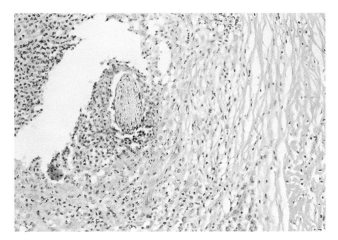

Figure 9-6   Free hair in the tissue, with surrounding inflammation and fibrosis. (×100.)

the overwhelmingly preferred location, but in the study by George et al,[2] 3% of those affected had parietal lesions.

HISTOLOGY

A dense follicular and perifollicular inflammatory infiltrate is seen early (Figures 9-5 to 9-7). As noted, this inflammation begins somewhere between the insertion of the arrector pili muscle to just above the connection of the sebaceous duct (deep infundibular or isthmian level).[4] Later, presumably after follicular rupture, necrotic tissue and fragments of hair (often best seen with polarization) are found. Transepidermal elimination of necrotic tissue and hair fragments is characteristic,[5] especially if a crusted umbilical papule is biopsied. Prominent fibrosis occurs later.

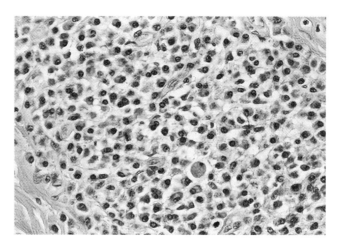

Figure 9-7   Cellular infiltrate with many plasma cells. (×400.)

DIFFERENTIAL DIAGNOSIS

The diagnosis is usually obvious. Very rarely, papular sarcoidosis can mimic acne keloidalis nuchae.

TREATMENT

Medical Intervention

The hair should be allowed to grow long in the affected area. Some patients staunchly resist this advice because they are fond of the shaved look. Mechanical irritation by a tight collar should be avoided if possible, although some patients find this difficult because of the professional attire required by their work. The patient should be encouraged not to pick or squeeze lesions.

To control the infectious component, either topical (e.g., clindamycin, erythromycin) or oral (e.g., Keflex 250 mg qid) antibiotics should be given. Benzoyl peroxide is usually best avoided because it can bleach the hair. If any pustules are present, bacterial culture should be done to ensure that an appropriate antibiotic is being used. Hair oils should be avoided. Sometimes the inflammatory and/or infectious component resists these measures. It may be that previous scarring has created pockets of infection that are not fully exposed to therapy. Rotation of antibiotics, reculture, and even a course of isotretinoin may be needed. A sterile inflammatory component may respond to one of the tetracyclines (e.g., tetracycline 500 mg bid, minocycline 100 mg bid).

Once any infection has been controlled, the keloids may be treated by injection with Kenalog 10 to 40 mg/cc every 4 weeks. Either a 25-gauge needle or the dermajet may be used. A facial mask or other such protection should be worn by the physician while injecting. Usually, the lower concentration is used initially, and injections are performed every 4 weeks. If no adverse effects are seen (e.g., hypopigmentation, atrophy of normal skin), the concentration may be increased up to 40 mg/cc. Traditionally, physicians avoid giving more than 20 mg total per 4 weeks. Topical steroids (usually class I or II) may be used between visits.

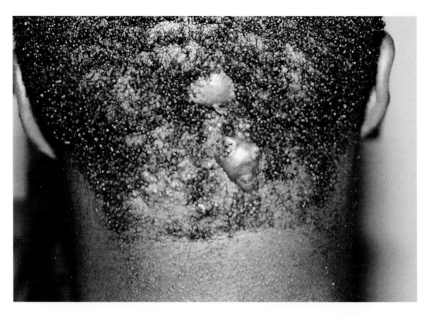

Figure 9-8   Recurrence of keloids after CO_2 laser surgery was performed on this patient 4 months earlier. The two large nodules represent recurrent disease that is larger than the initial lesions.

SURGICAL INTERVENTION

If significant shrinkage of lesions is not obtained after 3 to 4 injections, a surgical approach may be tried. Some success may be achieved by shaving lesions flat, followed by postoperative intralesional corticosteroid therapy (e.g., 20 to 40 mg/cc every 2 to 4 weeks) combined with a potent topical steroid (e.g., clobetasol) and an oral antibiotic.[6] However, this approach is not nearly as reliable as those that remove diseased tissue to the subfollicular level. In fact, larger keloids may result.

Small papular lesions may be removed via punch biopsy (e.g., using a hair transplant punch down to fibrous tissue). The CO_2 laser may be used effectively if removal is carried out to a subfollicular depth[7] (Figure 9-8). Healing should be allowed to occur through secondary intention. The placement of grafts does not provide substantial cosmetic benefit and may inhibit the contraction that is desired to reduce the final scar. Patients should be informed that healing may take up to 6 weeks. Occasionally, intralesional application of Kenalog may be needed if any excessive scarring is seen during the healing process.

Definitive therapy of severe disease with large keloids and sinus tracts is obtained by surgical debulking. The best results in one study[8] were achieved with a horizontal, elliptical excision, including the posterior hairline down to muscle fascia or the deep subcutaneous tissue (Figure 9-9). The wound may be allowed to heal by secondary intention. Alternatively, primary closure after wide undermining for smaller lesions and the use of a tissue expander inserted above the keloid for larger lesions may be done. It cannot be overemphasized that any excision or destruction must be carried out to the subfollicular depth. If any portion of the hair follicle is left, recurrence is common and/or wound contraction is not as great. The patient should be informed that the goal of such therapy is an asymptomatic but alopetic scar.

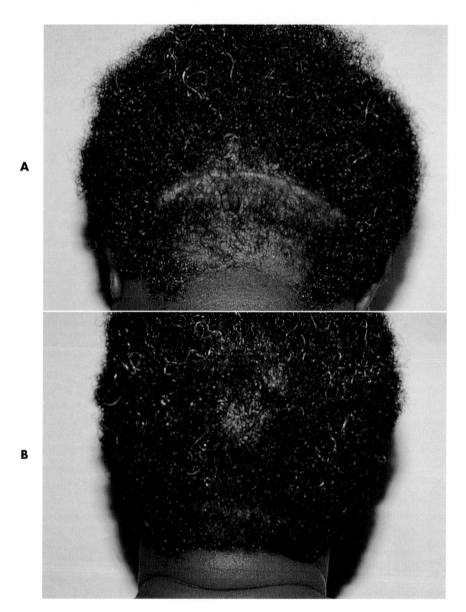

Figure 9-9   Acne keloidalis nuchae after surgical excision. **A,** A horizontal, elliptical excision to remove the diseased tissue has been made. **B,** Note how well the hair covers the defect.

Radiation therapy of the base of the wound to ablate any persistent inflammation has been advocated, but concerns about use of radiation in a young patient with a benign disease make most shy away from this modality. Treatment with oral retinoids has not been impressive.

REFERENCES

1. Dinehart SM et al: Acne keloidalis in women, *Cutis* 44:250-252, 1989.
2. George AO et al: Clinical, biochemical and morphologic features of acne keloidalis in a black population, *Int J Dermatol* 32:714-716, 1993.
3. Dinehart SM et al: Acne keloidalis: a review, *J Dermatol Surg Oncol* 15:642-647, 1989.
4. Herzberg AJ et al: Acne keloidalis: transverse microscopy, immunohistochemistry and electron microscopy, *Am J Dermatopathol* 12:109-121, 1990.
5. Goette DK, Berger TG: Acne keloidalis nuchae: a transepithelial elimination disorder, *Int J Dermatol* 26:442-444, 1987.
6. Harland CC et al: Combined surgical and medical treatment of acne keloidalis, *Br J Dermatol* (abstract) (suppl 44), 131:47-48, 1994.
7. Kantor GHR, Ratz JL, Wheeland RG: Treatment of acne keloidalis nuchae with carbon dioxide laser, *J Am Acad Dermatol* 14:263-267, 1986.
8. Glenn MJ, Bennett RG, Kelly AP: Acne keloidalis nuchae: treatment with excision and second-intention healing, *J Am Acad Dermatol* 33:243-246, 1995.

Chapter 10

Dermatosis Papulosa Nigra

Gary M. White

*D*ermatosis papulosa nigra is a fancy name for a common and entirely benign condition experienced by many black adults. It is characterized by growth on the face and neck of multiple pigmented papules that histologically resemble seborrheic keratoses. Women seem to be more commonly affected than men, and there is often a positive family history. Hairston, Reed, and Derbes[1] found the incidence of dermatosis papulosa nigra to be 35% in adult black patients. Of those those with facial lesions, 24% also had lesions on their bodies. In another study,[2] darker-skinned patients had a higher incidence, and the number of lesions peaked for patients in their 60s. Prepubescent children may rarely be affected.[3]

CLINICAL

Multiple pigmented papules, flat or filiform, on the face and neck of a darker-skinned person are characteristic of dermatosis papulosa nigra (Figure 10-1). Lesions are well demarcated and are typically 1 to 5 mm in size. Favored areas include the malar eminences and temples. Lesions on the trunk may also occur. This condition is in no way harmful, but lesions may be very annoying, catching on jewelry or even obstructing vision.

HISTOLOGY

The microscopic pattern of dermatosis papulosa nigra is the same as that of a seborrheic keratosis.[1]

TREATMENT

Treatment may be indicated for cosmetic reasons or if any specific lesion is particularly bothersome. Snipping the lesion at the base is simple and effective. It may be done relatively painlessly without anesthesia if the base is small (e.g., ≤2 mm). Otherwise, the area may be infiltrated locally with lidocaine before removal. Another very effective method of removal is electrodesiccation at a very low setting after administra-

---

The lesions should not *be frozen because hypopigmentation may result.*

tion of local anesthesia (Figure 10-2). A piece of gauze can then be used to wipe away the lesion. Aluminum chloride or Monsel's solution may be applied for hemostasis after either procedure. The lesions should *not* be frozen because hypopigmentation may result.

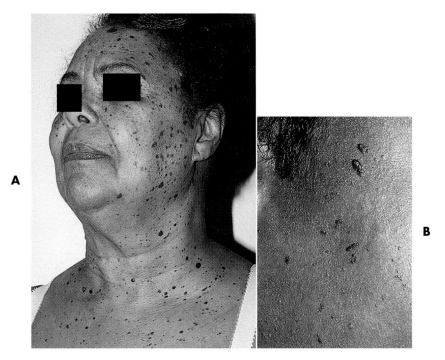

Figure 10-1   Dermatosis papulosa nigra. This woman was greatly bothered by the many brown papules on her face and neck.

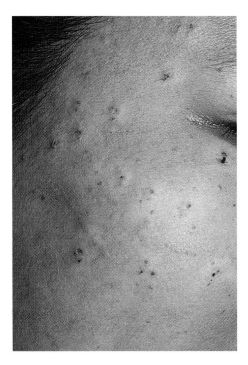

Figure 10-2   Dermatosis papulosa nigra after light electrodesiccation.

REFERENCES

1. Hairston MA, Reed RJ, Derbes VJ: Dermatosis papulosa nigra, *Arch Dermatol* 89:655-658, 1964.
2. Grimes PE et al: Dermatosis papulosa nigra, *Cutis* 32:385-392, 1983.
3. Babapour R, Leach J, Levy H: Dermatosis papulosa nigra in a young child, *Pediatr Dermatol* 10:356-358, 1993.

Keloids

Bernett L. Johnson, Jr.

K eloids are shiny, hyperpigmented, thick, raised, hard, papulonodular plaques and tumors.

INCIDENCE

The true incidence of keloids is unknown. They occur with greatest frequency in the second and third decades. Both sexes are equally affected. Keloids are known to occur with greater frequency in black skin, but they have been found in all races.[1,2]

Keloids are known to occur with greater frequency in black skin, but they have been found in all races.

ETIOLOGY

The etiology of the keloid is unknown. It is thought that trauma plays a major role, although keloids have been reported to develop without trauma (spontaneous keloids). The role of trauma may be the initiating factor in a fibroblast mast cell interaction whereby the mast cell produces fibroblast growth factor that prolongs the growth phase and allows for excessive growth.[3] Keloids occur after surgical procedures, and by definition extend beyond the area included in the procedure.

CLINICAL MANIFESTATIONS

Clinically, keloids are very dense and hard (Figure 11-1). The borders are hyperpigmented, whereas the centers are lighter. Although the borders are usually smooth, they may have finger or clawlike extensions. Keloids can be painful or pruritic or both. It is these symptoms, as well as their appearance, that initiate the patient's visit to the physician. Keloids can be found on any site, and have even been seen on the cornea. The most common sites are the earlobes, upper back, midchest, and shoulders (Figure 11-2). Specific variations of keloids that are seen in black men include pseudofolliculi-

---

Keloids can be found on any site, and have even been seen on the cornea.

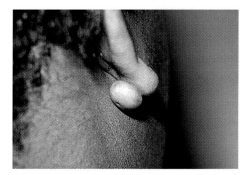

Figure 11-1 Firm, hard keloid of the ear lobe, a very common site for development.

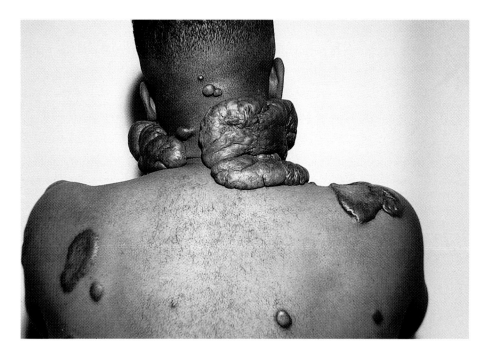

Figure 11-2 Giant keloids of the neck, shoulders, and back.

tis and acne keloidalis. These follicular keloidal growths are associated with and induced by hair that is extrafollicular and treated as if it were a foreign body. These conditions are covered in detail in other sections of the book.

HISTOLOGY

Histologically, keloids show epidermal thinning and atrophy (Figures 11-3 and 11-4). The dermis is replaced by a fibrocellular reaction in which thick, eosinophilic, hyalinized, sclerotic collagen bundles are imbedded. These sclerotic collagen bodies are the hallmark of keloids. The fibrocellular reaction is separated from the normal epidermis but can extend into the epidermis in thin, fingerlike strands of fibrous reaction. This reaction can extend into and replace the subcutis. The cells seen in the inflammatory fibrocellular reaction are lymphocytes, fibroblasts, histiocytes, and mast cells.

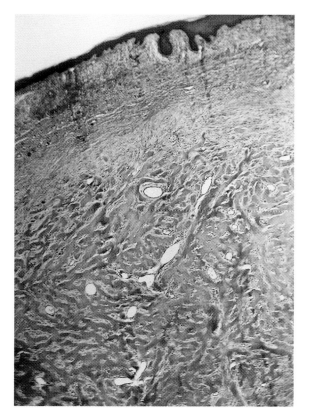

Figure 11-3 A fibrocellular reaction in the dermis with sclerotic collagen bodies embedded in the fibrous matrix. (×20.)

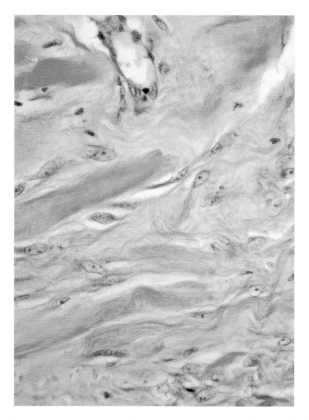

Figure 11-4 Higher-power image of the collagen bodies, a hallmark of keloids. (×100.)

The clinical differential diagnoses of keloids are dermatofibrosarcoma protuberans, squamous cell carcinoma (SCC), and keloidal deep fungal infections. Differentiation from a "hypertrophic scar" may be difficult.

TREATMENT

The treatment of keloids is as frustrating for the patient as it is for the physician and is often futile. Treatment options are covered in Chapters 22 and 23.

REFERENCES

1. Berman B, Bielley HC: Keloids, *J Am Acad Dermatol* 33(1):117, 1995.
2. Datubo-Brown DD: Keloids: a review of the literature, *Br J Plast Surg* 43(1):70, 1990.
3. Johnson BL, Kelly P, Lavker R: Mast cell interactions in keloids (personal communication).

Chapter 12

Pseudofolliculitis Barbae

Gary M. White

Pseudofolliculitis barbae is a common condition of the beard area in black men who shave closely.[1,2] *Razor bumps* is a common term used by the lay public for this condition. The underlying process is tissue damage and foreign body response to the patient's own hair. The most effective treatment is for the patient to grow a beard.

EPIDEMIOLOGY

Pseudofolliculitis barbae primarily affects adult black men. The incidence in black men who shave ranges widely from 10% to 83%. Black or white women who shave in the axillary or pubic region may be similarly affected. One hirsute, black, female patient who shaved in the submental region developed it there as well. A clinical association between pseudofolliculitis barbae and acne keloidalis nuchae has been noted, and implies an underlying predisposition to both disorders. Pseudofolliculitis barbae is a common problem in black men who are members of the military, where a close shave is standard.[2]

ETIOLOGY

The hair follicle in the black patient is curved (Figure 12-1) and the whisker is flattened, which results in a curved whisker. Histologic sections show that the whisker forms a nearly perfect circular arc in the dermis and exits the skin almost parallel to the surface. Because these hairs hug the surface, many are missed during shaving; if they are cut, a very sharp point results. Invariably, some of these whiskers will grow the few millimeters necessary to complete the extracutaneous arc and reenter the skin. The whisker's sharp tip aids in the puncturing of the skin surface, which in this scenario is called *extrafollicular penetration*. Swelling and inflammation in the form of a neutrophilic foreign-body response develops. Papules and pustules in close proximity to the follicle result.

The hair follicle in the black patient is curved and the whisker is flattened, which results in a curved whisker.

Intrafollicular (or transfollicular) penetration occurs when the hair whose tip is below the skin's surface penetrates the follicular wall as it grows. Such a short hair is created by pulling the skin taught while shaving, by plucking hairs, or by using a shaving system that lifts the hair before cutting. Subsequent shaving often cuts or traumatizes the papules, causing more swelling and making the whisker more likely to dig into the papule. Bacterial infection may occur secondarily, but is not the primary process.

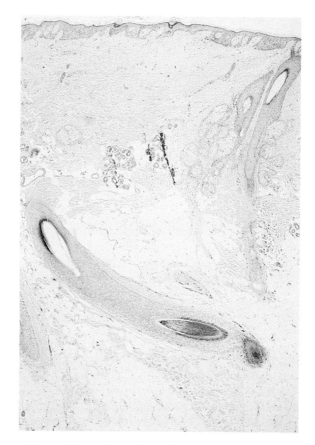

Figure 12-1   Curved hair follicle in a black patient.

CLINICAL

Clinical examination of the patient shows multiple symmetric, inflammatory papules, many with short whiskers penetrating their bases (Figure 12-2). These papules are always found in close proximity (e.g., 1 to 3 mm) to a whisker. The submandibular area and neck are common locations. For unknown reasons, the mustache area tends to be spared. Pustules and occasional abscesses are seen, but as noted above, any infection is a secondary event. Papules readily bleed with shaving. Postinflammatory hyperpigmentation and even keloid formation can develop. In long-standing disease, the whiskers can create grooves in the skin (Figure 12-3). The whisker then lies below the surface of the skin in the groove and is hard to cut by the usual shaving techniques. Sometimes a superficial, criss-cross pattern can result. Once these grooves have formed, the condition becomes very difficult to treat.

In long-standing disease, the whiskers can create grooves in the skin. Sometimes a superficial, criss-cross pattern can result.

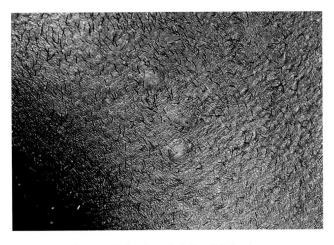

Figure 12-2   Pseudofolliculitis barbae.

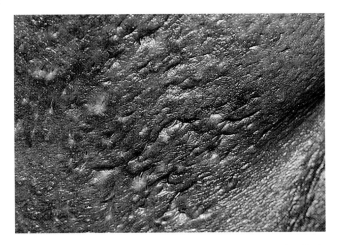

Figure 12-3   Typical shallow scars of pseudofolliculitis barbae with whiskers lying in the groove.

HISTOLOGY

The whisker traumatizes the epidermis either through extrafollicular or intrafollicular penetration. A foreign-body response ensues, causing dermal abscesses and epidermal microabscesses.

DIFFERENTIAL DIAGNOSIS

The diagnosis is rarely in question, and biopsy is generally not needed. Acne of the face presents with comedones as well as papules and pustules. A true bacterial folliculitis is rarely chronic and does not scar like pseudofolliculitis barbae. In one unusual case, firm, keloidlike papules within a man's pseudofolliculitis barbae represented sarcoidosis.[3]

TREATMENTS

Hair-Releasing Procedures

Trapped hairs are a constant source of irritation and are less accessible to any shaving technique. Thus hair-releasing procedures as outlined below should be performed in the first month of growing a beard or in conjunction with the use of chemical depilatories, razors, or electric shavers or clippers. The typical approach is to instruct the patient to use a toothpick and a magnifying mirror to gently extract the hairs. A sterile needle may be needed if the hair is completely buried. Patients should not pluck hairs. Other approaches include hair-releasing kits sold over the counter, brushing the beard, and cleansing with a washcloth or Buf-Puf.

Wearing a Beard

Growing a beard is curative. If the patient's work, social, and personal situations allow, immediate cessation of shaving is recommended. Over the following month, the patient should release any trapped hairs every few days. Even if the patient is unable to release all the hairs, the natural growth of the whisker will eventually create enough tension in the "coil" that it will pop out on its own. The doctor should always ask about the patient's work situation and specifically whether the patient needs a letter addressed to his employer excusing the patient from shaving. Of note, cessation of shaving may be employed for 3 to 4 weeks to release all hairs and reduce inflammation before beginning any of the following procedures (Box 12-1).

The doctor should always ask about the patient's work situation and specifically whether the patient needs a letter addressed to his employer excusing the patient from shaving.

Chemical Depilatories

If a close shave is necessary, several approaches may be tried. The patient may do well using a depilatory. Those with barium sulfide (e.g., Magic Shave) or calcium thioglycolate (e.g., Magic Shave Gold Powder) should be used every 2 to 4 days. Some products are powders that must be mixed, whereas others are ready to use. The product is applied to a portion of the beard for a prescribed number of minutes. It is removed with a blunt instrument such as a wooden tongue depressor. The face is then washed several times with cool to lukewarm water. Longer treatments than recommended can cause significant irritation of the skin (or even a chemical burn). Some ex-

---

Box 12-1   Treatment Options for Pseudofolliculitis Barbae

Grow a beard
Chemical depilatory (barium sulfide or calcium thioglycolate) every 2 to 4 days*
Clipper*
Electric shaver*
Razor*

---

*A hair-releasing procedure must be used adjunctively.

perts have recommended not washing the face before using a depilatory, to allow the face's natural oils to act as a protective barrier. Hydrocortisone 1% cream may be applied after depilatory use. The main disadvantages to chemical depilatories are their objectionable odor and the irritation that they can cause. One advantage is that because the depilatory works by dissolving disulfide bonds, the remaining hair tip is feathered and less able to pierce the intact skin.

Razors

Various razors are available and marketed for use by patients with pseudofolliculitis barbae. The foil-guard razor has been studied[4] and its use was found to be beneficial. It contains a single stainless-steel blade that is buffered from the patient's skin by a serrated foil guard. Alternatively, an adjustable razor may be used, with the patient selecting the very lowest settings to avoid a close shave. Twin blades should not be used because they may lift the whisker, cut it, and allow it to retract below the skin surface. This can lead to intrafollicular penetration.

When any razor blade is used, the patient must (1) not apply significant pressure, (2) shave with the grain, (3) shave any given area only once, and (4) not use the free hand to pull the skin taut. Putting the free hand in one's pocket is a helpful hint. Finally, preshave measures used to soften the whiskers are important. A shaving cream should be applied and allowed to sit for 2 to 5 minutes before shaving. Some recommend a second application.[2] This long presoak softens the whiskers, making one pass of the razor more effective.

There is a tendency for some patients to shave infrequently. The danger here is that the whisker may have enough time to form an arc and circle back into the skin. Thus shaving is recommended at least every 3 days.[5]

Electric Shavers

Alternatively, the use of an electric shaver may be an improvement over a blade for many. The three-headed rotary electric razor can produce good results.[6] It is important to use the electric razor in a circular motion with a "gentle hand." If the patient has a significant beard, the clipper portion of the shaver should be used first to remove the bulk of the whiskers.

Clippers

Electric clippers are advocated by a variety of authors as an ideal approach to therapy.[7,8] Shaving may be done daily, leaving about a 1-mm "stubble" that in the black patient is usually less noticeable than in the white patient.

Other Interventions

Inflammation is not caused by infection, but may be aggravated by it. Thus topical clindamycin or erythromycin applied twice daily may be tried when inflammation is significant. In an 8-week study by Perricone,[9] 8% glycolic acid lotion applied twice daily was dramatically more effective than placebo at reducing the papules and pustules of the face and neck. Tretinoin has been recommended,[10] but not proved effective in a placebo-controlled trial.

Surgical depilations, where the skin is peeled back and the hair roots are clipped, have a significant complication rate. Finally, electrolysis is to be avoided because the curved follicle is difficult to destroy, and significant scarring may occur.

REFERENCES

1. Strauss JS, Kligman AM: Pseudofolliculitis of the beard, *Arch Dermatol Syphilol* 74:533-542, 1956.
2. Coquilla BH, Lewis CW: Management of pseudofolliculitis barbae, *Mil Med* 160:263-269, 1995.
3. Norton SA, Chesser RS: Scar sarcoidosis in pseudofolliculitis barbae, *Mil Med* 156:369-371, 1991.
4. Alexander AM: Evaluation of a foil-guarded shaver in the management of pseudofolliculitis barbae, *Cutis* 27:534-542, 1981.
5. Brauner GJ, Flandermeyer KL: Pseudofolliculitis barbae. II. Treatment, *Int J Dermatol* 16:520-525, 1977.
6. Garcia RL, Henderson R: The adjustable rotary electric razor in the control of pseudofolliculitis barbae, *J Assoc Mil Derm* 4:28, 1978.
7. Conte MS, Lawrence JE: Pseudofolliculitis barbae: no pseudoproblem, *JAMA* 241:53-54, 1979.
8. Brown LA: Pathogenesis and treatment of pseudofolliculitis barbae, *Cutis* 32:373-375, 1983.
9. Perricone NV: Treatment of pseudofolliculitis barbae with topical glycolic acid: a report of two studies, *Cutis* 52:232, 1993.
10. Kligman AM, Mills OH: Pseudofolliculitis of the beard and topically applied tretinoin, *Arch Dermatol* 107:551-552, 1973.

Chapter 13

Sarcoidosis

Bernett L. Johnson, Jr.

Sarcoidosis is a granulomatous disease of unknown etiology that affects patients with black skin with greater frequency and severity than any other ethnic group. In 1899 sarcoidosis was defined in the literature by Boeck as "multiple benign sarcoid of the skin," although in 1865 this disease had been recorded by Sir Jonathan Hutchinson as an iritis. Although sarcoidosis was thought of only as a cutaneous disease, in 1914 Schumann became aware of and defined the correlation of the cutaneous and systemic forms of sarcoidosis.[1]

Sarcoidosis is a granulomatous disease of unknown etiology that affects patients with black skin with greater frequency and severity than any other ethnic group.

INCIDENCE

The incidence of sarcoid varies from 200 cases per 100,000 population to 20 cases per 100,000 population. Studies comparing black and white populations show the incidence to be 7.6 cases per 100,000 population for whites and 81.8 cases per 100,000 population for blacks, with a ratio of black to white patients reportedly reaching as high as 18:1. Black females are affected twice as often as black men.[1,2]

ETIOLOGY

There have been numerous attempts to isolate an organism from the tissue of sarcoidal patients, but no bacterial, fungal, or viral organisms have been identified. There is also a close similarity in the histology of sarcoidosis to that of granulomas produced by zirconium and beryllium, but these elements are not a factor in this disease. There is no familial or inherited incidence in sarcoidosis.

CLINICAL MANIFESTATIONS

Cutaneous and systemic manifestations are the hallmark of sarcoidosis. In patients with black skin, sarcoidosis is a more severe disease, although the incidence of pulmonary adenopathy—the usual signal event in this disease—is slightly less in black patients.[2] The cutaneous manifestations of sarcoidosis in black skin are strikingly different from those of other ethnic groups. The clinical forms of sarcoidosis seen almost exclusively in black skin are addressed below.

Cutaneous and systemic manifestations are the hallmark of sarcoidosis. In patients with black skin sarcoidosis is a more severe disease.

Ichthyosis

In icthyosiform manifestations of sarcoidosis, the skin is dry, scaly, and ashy white, without the presence of papules or nodules (Figures 13-1 and 13-2).

Hypopigmented Macule

The hypopigmented macular form of sarcoidosis is referred to as *"Philadelphia"* sarcoid because it is commonly seen in that city, to the exclusion of the rest of the country. The lesion is macular, hypopigmented or depigmented, and without substance when compressed (Figure 13-3).

Scarring Alopecia

A scarring alopecia of the type seen in lupus, fungus, hot comb, or lichen planus is seen in sarcoidosis. The usually distinctive, red-brown papules or nodules are not seen, but granulomas are found on histologic sections (Figure 13-4).

Ulcers

Sarcoidal ulcerations occur in the skin and are frequently found on the lower extremities. The ulcers themselves are not distinctive. Granulomas are found on histology (Figure 13-5).

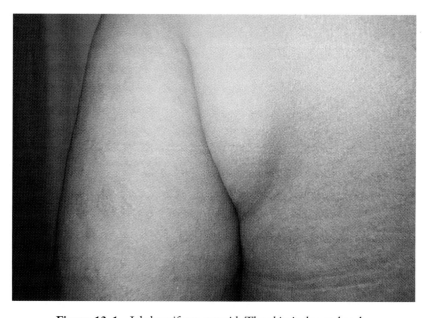

Figure 13-1 Ichthyosiform sarcoid. The skin is dry and scaly.

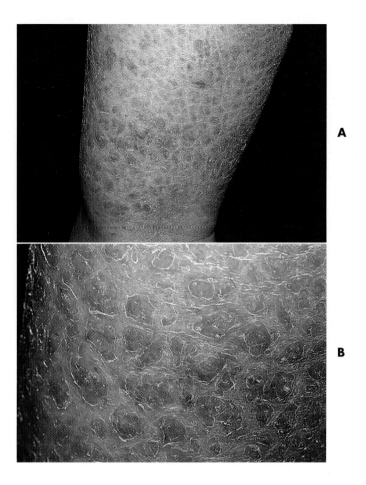

Figure 13-2 Sarcoidosis presenting as ichthyosis.

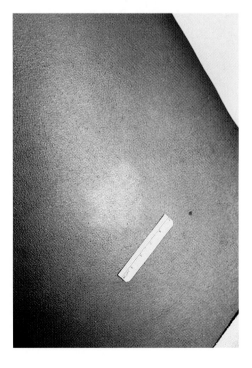

Figure 13-3 Hypopigmented, macular (Philadelphia) sarcoid.

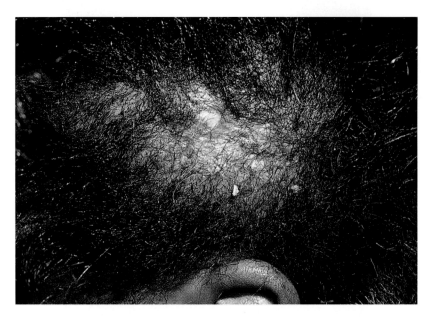

Figure 13-4 Alopecia of sarcoidosis.

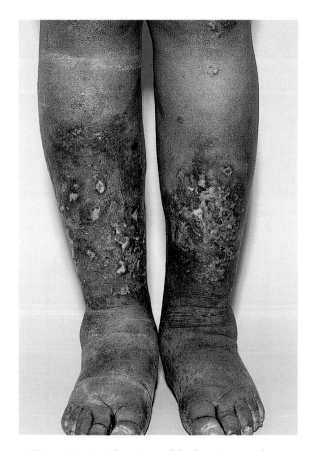

Figure 13-5 Ulceration of the legs in sarcoidosis.

Keloids

Keloidal sarcoids are cutaneous lesions that are firm, shiny, dome-shaped, and hard (Figure 13-6).

Annuli

Annular configurations of violaceous papules and/or nodules are also manifestations of sarcoidosis. These lesions resemble granuloma annulare, pityriasis rosea, and annular lichen planus (Figure 13-7).

Discoid Lupuslike Lesions

Discoid lupuslike lesions of sarcoidosis are annular, atrophic lesions with raised, pigmented borders and atrophic, hypopigmented centers (Figure 13-8).

Verrucae

Hypertrophic, hyperkeratotic lesions resembling verrucae may also be preset.

Black patients also have the more classic beaded, red-brown papules on the nasal rim or eyelid margins (Figure 13-9). Lupus pernio and erythema nodosum, conditions commonly seen in nonblack skin, are rare in black skin.[3]

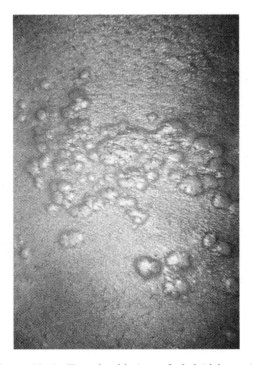

Figure 13-6   Firm, hard lesions of a keloidal sarcoid.

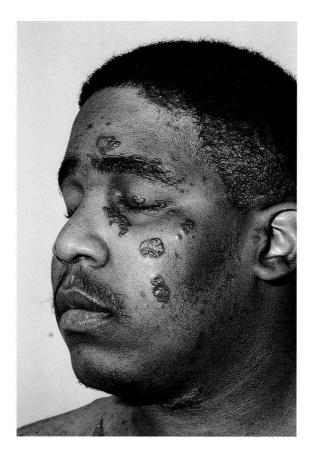

Figure 13-7   Annular, violaceous, confluent papules.

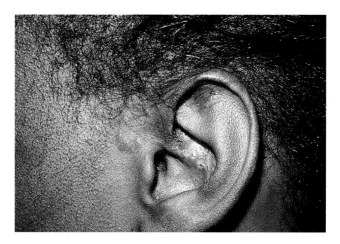

Figure 13-8   Discoid lupuslike sarcoid with ear lesions.

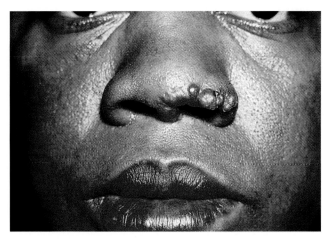

Figure 13-9 Typical beaded, red-brown papules of the alar rim.

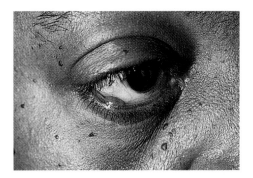

Figure 13-10 Conjunctival granuloma of sarcoid.

SYSTEMIC DISEASE

Black patients exhibit a wide variety of systemic diseases associated with sarcoidosis. Systemic involvement includes the following types.

Lupus pernio and erythema nodosum, conditions commonly seen in nonblack skin, are rare in black skin.

Ocular Conditions

Lacrimal gland enlargement, granulomas on the conjunctiva (Figure 13-10), uveitis, chorioretinitis, and posterior chamber involvement are all ocular conditions common in sarcoidosis. Others include neovascularization, obstructive glaucoma, and disk edema.

Musculoskeletal Conditions

Myositis, muscular atrophy or hypertrophy, and cystic bone change are common in sarcoidosis.

Other Systemic Involvement

Other systemic manifestations of sarcoidosis include changes in bone marrow (17%), renal involvement (calculi), granulomatous liver disease, cardiac conduction defects, and cardiac granulomas. The lymphatic system may experience hilar or peripheral adenopathy. In the endocrine system, there may be hypothalamus and pituitary involvement with related symptoms or granulomas may be found in other major endocrine glands without symptoms.

LABORATORY ABNORMALITIES

Laboratory abnormalities common in sarcoidosis include hypercalcemia (secondary to increased absorption), hypercalciuria, elevated angiotensin-converting enzyme levels, increased urinary and serum lysozyme levels, increased B_2 macroglobulin, and increased serum collagenase.

ASSOCIATED DISEASES

Diseases associated with sarcoidosis include progressive systemic sclerosis, systemic lupus erythematosus, prophyria cutanea tarda, IgA deficiency, primary cirrhosis, and T-cell lymphoma. Patients with sarcoidosis also exhibit significant cellular and humoral immunity (Box 13-1).

HISTOLOGY

The histologic features of sarcoidosis in all skin types are the same except for the presence of pigment in black, Asian, and some Hispanic skin. All show epithelioid granulomas in the dermis that are composed of collections of epithelioid histiocytes and

---

Box 13-1   Immunologic Abnormalities in Sarcoidosis

Cell Mediated
Depressed circulating T cells
Anergy to skin test
Depressed lymphocyte transformation
Decreased neutrophil phagocytosis
Suppressor macrophages in blood
Leukotactic dysfunction of monocytes and polycytes

Humoral
Polyclonal hypergammaglobulinemia
False positive serologic test for syphilis (STS)
Circulating immune complexes
Decreased ability to opsonize yeast
Increased serum-free light chains

surrounded and infiltrated by lymphocytes, with the latter becoming more scarce as the granulomas age (Figures 13-11 and 13-12). Granulomas may show necrosis, although this is not the usual finding. Inclusions such as Schaumann's bodies (calcium carbonate/phosphate and iron) and asteroid bodies (lipoprotein) can be found in the granulomas. Lipomucoprotein granules, IgG, and C_3 can be found in the granulomas.

The histologic features of sarcoidosis in all skin types are the same except for the presence of pigment in black, Asian, and some Hispanic skin.

Figure 13-11   Epithelioid cell granulomas in the dermis ($\times$40.)

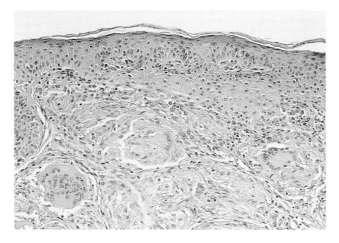

Figure 13-12   High power image of dermal granulomas. There is sparse epidermal pigment in this hypopigmented sarcoid. ($\times$200.)

TREATMENT

The successful treatment of sarcoidosis is difficult; spontaneous resolution of acute disease occurs in 70% to 80% of patients. The mainstay of therapy is the use of corticosteroids, which may be administered orally, intralesionally, intramuscularly, and as eye drops. A host of other agents have been used with varying success and include the following:

Allopurinol	Oxyphenbutazone
Antimalarials	PABA
Azothioprine	Retinoids
Chlorambucil	Tetracycline
Cyclosporine	Thalidomide
Indomethacin	Thymic humoral factor
Levamisole	TP-5 (synthetic pentapeptide)
Methotrexate	Transfer factor

REFERENCES

1. Kerdel FA, Moschella SL: Sarcoidosis, *J Am Acad Dermatol* 11:1, 1984.
2. Sartwell SE: Racial differences in sarcoidosis, *Ann NY Acad Sci* 278:368, 1976.
3. Veien NK, Stahl D, Brodthagen H: Cutaneous sarcoid in caucasians, *J Am Acad Dermatol* 16:534, 1987.

Chapter 14

Vitiligo

Bernett L. Johnson, Jr.

INCIDENCE AND ETIOLOGY

Vitiligo is a disorder of pigment loss of unknown etiology.[1,2] The appearance of vitiligo is striking in patients with dark skin. Although the incidence in these patients appears greater, the actual incidence is approximately 1% to 2% of the world's population—about 50 million persons. Males and females are equally affected. Vitiligo may occur at any age but most commonly occurs in the first to third decades. Congenital cases have been described. About one fourth of the cases occur before the age of 10; the remainder occur before the age of 40. There is a positive family history in about one third of the cases.

Vitiligo may occur at any age, but most commonly occurs in the first to third decades.

Although the exact cause of vitiligo is unknown, autoimmunity is the most widely accepted cause. Credence is given to this theory because of the association of vitiligo with other autoimmune diseases such as diabetes, thyroid disease, pernicious anemia, and collagen vascular diseases. There is often a history of severe sunburn before the development of vitiliginous lesions, although sunburn has not proved to be a causative agent and would not seem to be because sunlight is used as a part of many treatment regimens. Another proposed cause of vitiligo is self-destruction during the melanin production process caused by free radical production or cell wall sensitization. The sensitized cell is not recognized by the body's immune system and is destroyed. There is a form of vitiligo whose cause is known. Toxic vitiligo is caused by chemicals and was seen commonly in the rubber industry where monobenzyl ether of hydroquinone was used.

CLINICAL MANIFESTATION

Vitiligo starts with the sudden onset of white patches in the skin. The most common sites for the development of these patches are the hands, feet, genitalia, and face (periocular and perioral) (Figures 14-1 to 14-3). The clinical manifestations have been divided into three types: (1) generalized, (2) segmental, and (3) focal. The segmental type often follows a dermatome or affects one leg or arm. It is the most difficult type to repigment and ceases progression after 1 year. Onset is in childhood. Vitiligo is usually asymptomatic, although itching can be a frequent symptom. The patches of pig-

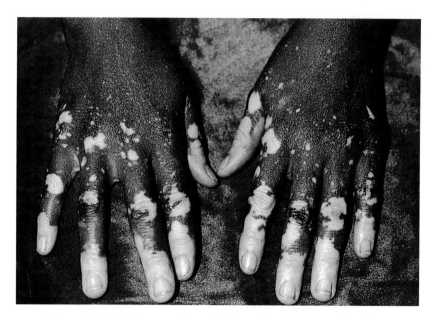

Figure 14-1   Depigmentation of the hands in a patient with vitiligo.

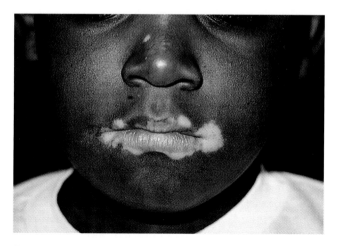

Figure 14-2   Perioral vitiligo.

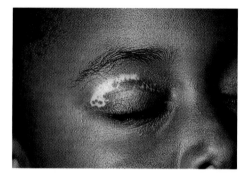

Figure 14-3   Periocular vitiligo with repigmentation.

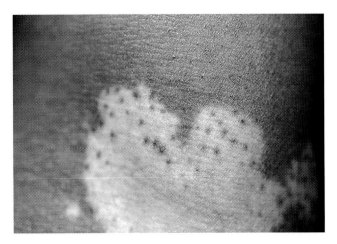

Figure 14-4 Vitiliginous spot with sharp, irregular borders.

ment loss are usually slowly progressive, and the course is unpredictable. There are cases in which the course is rapidly progressive, with total pigment loss occurring within several months. These cases are unusual and rare.

Vitiligo starts with the sudden onset of white patches in the skin.

The individual lesions of vitiligo are macular, without color, and have been described as "dead white." They have sharp but irregular borders that are often hyperpigmented (Figure 14-4).

The diagnosis of vitiligo is made based on the history and clinical presentation. There are no specific diagnostic tests, although biopsy is the most reliable diagnostic tool when done correctly. Two biopsies should be performed, one from the "lesion" and the other from an unaffected site. Specimens should be labeled as to site and submitted in formalin for analysis. Wood's light examination may be beneficial and is especially helpful in delineating the lesions in fair-skinned individuals. In very dark skin, however, the areas of pigment loss appear the same with or without the Wood's light.

HISTOLOGY

On routine sections, vitiligo is not striking or diagnostic. There may be absence of basal layer pigment or the presence of patchy pigment. In a recent review of many cases of vitiligo, a focally lichenoid inflammation was a consistent finding. In the area of lichenoid inflammation, melanocytes were atypical, and in many instances there was lymphocyte apposition to the altered melanocyte, similar to satellite cell necrosis as seen in graft versus host disease. Paired sections (involved and uninvolved areas), when stained for melanocytes or melanin, are the most helpful in diagnosing vitiligo histologically (Figure 14-5).

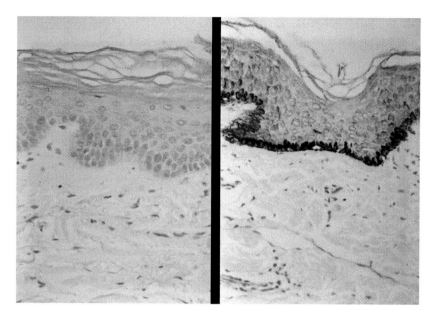

Figure 14-5 Vitiligo (left) and uninvolved skin (right). A Fontana stain showing pigment granules in the uninvolved skin and none in the vitiliginous skin. (×200.)

DIFFERENTIAL DIAGNOSIS

Differential diagnoses for vitiligo include tinea versicolor (positive KOH), pityriasis alba (Wood's light on pigment loss), postinflammatory hypopigmentation, morphea/scleroderma, and lichen sclerosus et atrophicus.

LABORATORY STUDIES

Before beginning therapy with psoralens and light, the physician should ensure that the following complete blood count (CBC), antinuclear antibody (ANA) tests, and studies are within normal limits: liver function tests (LFTs). A complete eye examination should be conducted, and the physician should rule out other contraindications to light therapy or sensitivity to psoralens. Extensive workups for other autoimmune diseases are usually unrewarding and not cost-effective. A good history and physical are still essential.

TREATMENT

The mainstays of the treatment of vitiligo are topical corticosteroids and PUVA in topical or systemic forms (Box 14-1). Treatment of vitiligo is often a year or more in duration because of the slow mobility of the melanocyte. Melanocytes that repopulate the vitiliginous areas come from two sources. Some come from the margins of the lesions, but most come from follicles. Melanocytes migrate to the epidermis around the follicle, accounting for the pigment dots seen during repigmentation (Figure 14-6). The follicles contain the melanocyte reservoir; if they are depigmented, repigmentation will not occur. Therapy is aimed at repigmenting the areas that have lost pigment and does not affect the cause of vitiligo or the development of new areas of pigment loss.

Box 14-1   Vitiligo Treatment Options

Repigmentation Agents
Topical corticosteroids
Topical PUVA
Systemic PUVA
Pseudocatalace and UVB*
Melagenina
Cyclosporine
UVB
Anapsos
Coal tar
Cyclophosphamide
Khellin
Vitamin E and PUVA
Clofazimine

Surgical Treatment
Punch and suction blister
Autologous grafts
Melanocyte cultures on dermabraded skin put into the blister space of a suction
    blister
Micropigmentation (tattooing)
Dermabrasion
Split-thickness grafts

Adjunctive Therapy
Sunscreens
Cosmetic covers
    Dermablend
    Covermark
Stains
    Chromalin
    Vitadye
    Walnut hull stain
Self-tanning lotions
Support groups
Psychologic support

Depigmentation Agent
Monobenzone (Benoquin)

Modified from Grimes PE: Vitiligo: current therapy, *Dermatol Clin* 11:325, 1993.
*From Schallreuter KU, et al: Treatment of vitiligo with a topical application of pseudocatalase and calcium
in combination with short-term UVB exposure: a case study on 33 patients, *Dermatology* 190:223, 1995.

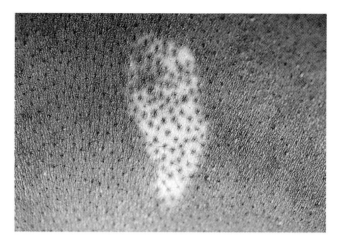

Figure 14-6   Repigmentation in a vitiligo lesion with many perifollicular pigment dots.

There have been no reports of an increased incidence of skin cancers after therapy for vitiligo.

The follicles contain the melanocyte reservoir; if they are depigmented, repigmentation will not occur.

Corticosteroids

All new patients should be given the option of being treated initially with topical corticosteroids if their involvement is 10% or less of their body surface area (BSA). Corticosteroids are effective in approximately 7% to 10% of cases. Mid- to high-potency strengths should be used. Corticosteroids can be used in all age groups and have been used in children as young as 2 years. Begin with the high-potency compounds and reduce the strength after about 1 to 2 months as pigment returns. When the sites have repigmented, a monthly maintenance dose of lower-potency compounds can be used. The side effects of steroid therapy are telangiectasis, striae, acne, and atrophy. The use of steroids on the eyelids and genitalia should be done with caution and for short periods, with careful monitoring and dispensing of only small amounts of medication. Steroid-based ointments work best.

Topical PUVA

Topical PUVA is recommended for those patients with involvement of 10% to 20% of BSA. It can be used in children over 2 years old. A solution of 0.1% Oxsoralen lotion or solution is applied to the affected sites and allowed to dry for 30 minutes. The patient is then exposed to UVA. The exposure depends on the skin type. Some general recommendations from the Oxsoralen package insert for use of PUVA are: type I skin—0.5 joules/cm^2; type II skin—1.0 joules/cm^2; type III skin—1.5 joules/cm^2; type IV skin—2.0 joules/cm^2; type V skin—2.5 joules/cm^2; and type VI skin—3.0 joules/cm^2. A summary of recommendations from the literature uses a lesser initial dose of UVA, beginning around 0.12 to 0.5 joules/cm^2. Some authors use a lesser dose initially for topical therapy than for systemic therapy. Skin types I and II always need lower initial doses.

After therapy, the treated areas are thoroughly washed with soap and water and covered with a sunscreen. The patient is instructed to avoid sun exposure. The patient should be treated weekly, and the light exposure slowly increased until erythema is maintained. Side effects of topical therapy are pruritus, blistering, diffuse tanning, xerosis, cataracts, burns, and skin cancer.

Systemic PUVA

Systemic PUVA is recommended for patients with greater than 20% BSA involvement. It is not recommended for use in children under 9 years of age. This therapy is based in antiquity and was noted to be effective as early as 1400 BC. Today's therapy, although it uses better drugs, is similar to that of earlier days. Oxsoralen Ultra (8-methoxsalen) 0.3 to 0.5 mg/kg is given to the patient 2 hours before light exposure. The recommended light exposures are the same as for topical therapy. The aim of therapy is to keep the skin pink without burning the patient. After therapy the patient is given wraparound sunglasses and told to wear them at all times indoors and outdoors; the sunglasses can be removed after 24 hours. The patient should be treated twice weekly, but never on consecutive days. The side effects of systemic therapy are nausea, vomiting, pruritus, xerosis, burns, cataracts, blistering, diffuse tanning, and skin cancer.

Depigmentation

Depigmentation is recommended when there is 50% or greater pigment loss, the patient will accept permanent pigment loss, and alternative therapies have failed. The affected areas of residual pigment should be treated with 10% to 20% monobenzone (Benoquin) twice daily. The initial therapy is from 1 to 3 months. As pigment fades, the frequency of application may be decreased. Repigmentation in some area does occur. Patients should avoid sun exposure, use a sunscreen on all areas, and avoid exposing other people to the medication because it will bleach their skin also.

Micropigmentation

The results of micropigmentation (tattooing) are not satisfactory. Risks include infection and transmission of disease. Color matching is very difficult. If the same color is placed at different depths in the tissue, the surface color will be different. Once the pigment is placed, it is not as easily removed as other tattoos.

Surgical Treatment

The surgical treatment of vitiligo is considered after medical treatment fails and is used mainly for cosmesis in small and localized areas. A detailed description of this and other medical therapies can be found in the literature and will not be detailed here.

Adunctive Therapy

Adjunctive therapy, although not considered major therapy, is nonetheless very important for the patient. Sunscreens are very important for protection of the vitiliginous skin. Cosmetic covers, either cosmetics or stains, are important to the patient and help return some sense of self by covering and hiding the pigment defects. This shields patients from questions and stares. Support groups and psychiatric care help treat the emotional aspects related to this condition. The treating physician can play a major role in the emotional healing by being compassionate and caring and by spending some time listening to the patient. This condition can be and often is devastating for people of color. In some cultures persons with vitiligo are outcasts and considered by many to be unclean; a woman with vitiligo may no longer be eligible for marriage. In our society, insurers of health care services consider the condition to be cosmetic and refuse to pay for care.

REFERENCES

1. Grimes PE: Vitiligo, *Dermatol Clin* 11(2):325, 1993.
2. Nordlund JJ, Halder RM, Grimes PE: Management of vitiligo, *Dermatol Clin* 11(1):27, 1993.

Chapter 15

Fox-Fordyce Disease

Gary M. White

Fox-Fordyce disease is caused by an obstruction of the apocrine sweat glands. Tens to hundreds of uniform, itchy papules of the axilla and other areas that contain apocrine glands result. A topical retinoid may be prescribed as treatment.

ETIOLOGY

Many things are known about Fox-Fordyce disease, but its cause remains unidentified. It seems fairly certain that a keratotic plug blocks the intraepidermal portion of the apocrine gland and prevents secretion.[1] A sweat-retention vesicle then results. Intraepidermal rupture follows—thus the term *apocrine miliaria*. Of note, obstruction of the apocrine gland alone, without rupture, does not result in the clinical changes of Fox-Fordyce disease. It is still not known, however, what causes the keratotic plug in the first place, why women are affected preferentially, and why hormonal changes influence the condition. Hormonal levels, when measured, are normal.

Fox-Fordyce disease seems to be caused by a keratotic plug that blocks the intraepidermal portion of the apocrine gland and prevents secretion. A functioning apocrine gland is a requirement of the disease, which is why it is rarely, if ever, seen before puberty.

EPIDEMIOLOGY

A functioning apocrine gland is a requirement of the disease, which is why it is rarely, if ever, seen before puberty. Women are affected 9:1 over men. Onset is usually from 13 to 35 years of age, although it has been reported as late as the postmenopausal years. Fox-Fordyce disease has been traditionally reported to occur preferentially in darker-skinned patients, although some authors believe that blacks and whites are equally predisposed. A brief survey of papers, including one by Shelley and Levy,[1] showed an approximately equal number of black and white patients reported (9 white, 8 black).

CLINICAL

The clinical appearance of Fox-Fordyce disease is uniformly distributed, pruritic, 2- to 3-mm, flesh-colored papules. Each papule is perifollicular and contains a central

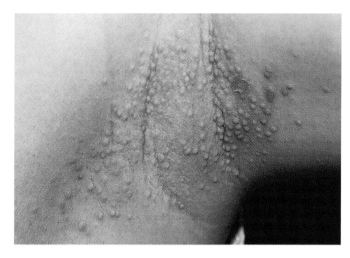

Figure 15-1   Fox-Fordyce disease in a Filipino woman. Note the uniformity of the papules and the sparsity of hair.

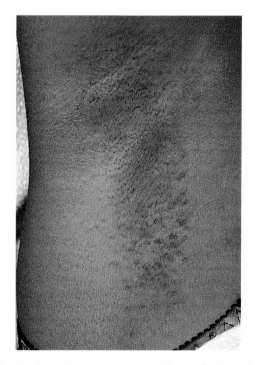

Figure 15-2   Fox-Fordyce disease in a teenage black girl. Note the sparsity of hair.

punctum or core. The central keratotic material may be expressed mechanically, and some physicians have noticed a milky fluid eminating from the papule. The distribution of these papules is restricted to the apocrine-bearing skin. The axilla (Figures 15-1 to 15-3) is most commonly affected, but the areola, groin, and perineum are potential sites. The intervening skin is normal. The papules are usually intensely pruritic, and the itching may vary with the menstrual cycle. Both premenstrual and menstrual exacerbation of the pruritus may occur. The hair in affected areas is sparse, and alopecia may even occur. The diminished presense of hair in most cases is probably unrelated to the

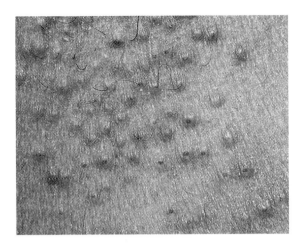

Figure 15-3   Many of the papules of Fox-Fordyce disease show a keratotic plug.

trauma of scratching. Significant regrowth of hair may occur after successful treatment. Some physicians have noted the axillary vault to be odorless, which probably reflects the cessation of apocrine secretion. Cases have been reported in which the patient's axillary body odor ceases with onset of the disease.

HISTOPATHOLOGY

A keratin plug blocks the intraepidermal portion of the apocrine duct. An intraepidermal sweat-retention vesicle results. This vesicle is the key diagnostic feature of Fox-Fordyce disease, because keratotic plugs alone are common in the axilla.[1] The proximal secretory portion of the vesicle may rupture, may be filled with periodic acid-Schiff (PAS)-positive material, or may be unaltered. Spongiosis, acanthosis, and/or the presence of an inflammatory infiltrate are changes that may be seen in the secretory portion of the apocrine duct.

DIFFERENTIAL DIAGNOSIS

The diagnosis of Fox-Fordyce disease is usually made clinically. Even in men, the many uniform-appearing and uniformly distributed flesh-colored papules in the axilla allow for an easy clinical diagnosis. A localized form of lichen simplex chronicus or follicular eczema could be considered, but the lack of lichenification, the normal appearance of the intervening skin, and the keratotic core of each papule allow for proper diagnosis.

TREATMENT

To dislodge the keratinaceous plug, a topical retinoid such as adapalene or tretinoin[2] may be used. Irritation may occur, and a mild topical steroid may also be used. The oral retinoid isotretinoin is effective,[3] but its routine use is impractical because long-term therapy is not justified, and the disease seems to recur after discontinuation. Birth control pills may[4] be helpful. Pregnancy may improve the eruption. Pasricha and Nayyar[5] used electrocautery successfully in two women. After local anesthesia, each lesion was electrocauterized to a depth of 3 to 4 mm. Several sittings were required, but both patients experienced complete relief for at least a year.

Clindamycin phosphate applied topically was rapidly successful in one case,[6] but it may have been the propylene glycol–containing vehicle that caused the improvement.

REFERENCES

1. Shelley WB, Levy EJ: Apocrine sweat retention in man: II. Fox-Fordyce disease (apocrine miliaria), *Arch Dermatol* 73:38-49, 1956.
2. Tkach JR: Tretinoin treatment of Fox-Fordyce disease, *Arch Dermatol* 115:1285, 1979.
3. Effendy I, Ossowski B, Haple R: Fox-Fordyce disease in a male patient: response to oral retinoid treatment, *Clin Exp Dermatol* 19:67-69, 1994.
4. Kronthal HL, Pomeranz JR, Sitomer G: Fox-Fordyce disease: treatment with an oral contraceptive, *Arch Dermatol* 91:243-245, 1965.
5. Pasricha JS, Nayyar KC: Fox-Fordyce disease in the post-menopausal period treated successfully with electrocoagulation, *Dermatologica* 147:271-273, 1973.
6. Feldman R et al: Fox-Fordyce disease: successful treatment with topical clindamycin in alcoholic propylene glycol solution, *Dermatology* 184:310-313, 1992.

Chapter 16

Papular Periorificial Dermatitis

Gary M. White

Granulomatous perioral dermatitis is a papular, inflammatory dermatosis found about the eyes, nostrils, and mouth in black children. It probably represents a papular variant of periorificial dermatitis in the darker-skinned patient. As with periorificial dermatitis, prior use of a potent topical steroid may predispose to this condition.

The appropriate name for this condition is under some dispute. The term *granulomatous perioral dermatitis* seems lacking because granulomas are not always seen histologically. Williams et al[1] proposed the term *FACE (Facial Afro-Caribbean Childhood Eruption)*, but Frieden and Esterly[2] object because of the occasional occurrence in other races and the occcasional extrafacial involvement. We prefer the term *papular periorificial dermatitis.*

CLINICAL

Children ages 3 to 11 are typically affected. Papules that are 1 to 3 mm, flesh-colored, and closely-grouped about the mouth, nose, and eyes in a darker-skinned child or adolescent are characterisitc of papular periorificial dermatitis (Figure 16-1). Most patients are black, but white children have been affected.[3] Extrafacial lesions may occasionally occur.[4] The eruption may wax and wane in intensity over time. Spontaneous resolution without scarring occurs; rarely, pinpoint atrophy may remain. One common feature of this disease is the often striking periorificial localization of the papules.

HISTOLOGY

Histologic analysis may show either a folliculitis or a perifollicular dermal granulomatous infiltrate surrounded by lymphocytes. In the initial report by Marten et al,[5] a granulomatous component was not described. It should be noted that Marten et al's series of 22 patients also differs from those of Frieden et al,[3] Miller and Shalita,[6] and Hansen, McTigue, and Esterly[4] by their lack of striking periorificial distributin (i.e., perioral, perinasal, and periorbital). Their patients almost always had involvement of the cheeks, helices of the ears, and upper eyelid.

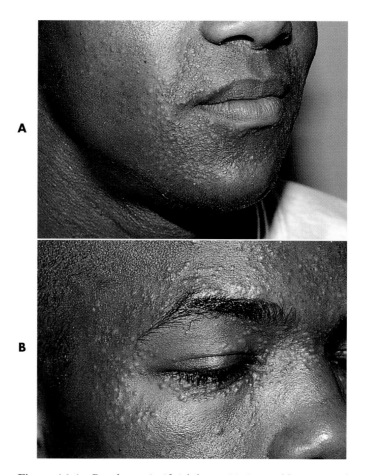

Figure 16-1   Papular periorificial dermatitis in an older teenage boy.

DIFFERENTIAL DIAGNOSIS

Diagnosis of papular periorificial dermatitis is usually made clinically. Granulomatous perioral dermatitis is differentiated from saroidosis by its lack of systemic involvement. A chest x-ray may be indicated in some cases.

TREATMENT

This disease responds poorly to treatment but undergoes spontaneous resolution, usually within 6 to 9 months. Interventions that have met with some success include metronidazole twice daily and oral erythromycin.

REFERENCES

1. Williams HC et al: FACE—facial Afro-Caribbean childhood eruption, *Clin Exp Dermatol* 15:163-166, 1990.
2. Frieden IJ, Esterly NB: In reply to "You say potato, we say potatoe," *Arch Dermatol* 130:114-115, 1994.

3. Frieden IJ et al: Granulomatous perioral dermatitis in children, *Arch Dermatol* 125:369-373, 1989.
4. Hansen KK, McTigue K, Esterly NB: Multiple facial, neck, and upper trunk papules in a black child, *Arch Dermatol* 128:1395, 1992.
5. Marten RH et al: An unusual papular and acneiform facial eruption in the Negro child, *Br J Dermatol* 91:435-438, 1974.
6. Miller SR, Shalita AR: Topical metronidazole gel (0.75%) for the treatment of perioral dermatitis in children, *J Am Acad Dermatol* 31:847-848, 1994.

Chapter 17

Exogenous Ochronosis

Gary M. White

Exogenous ochronosis is a rare condition in which dark papules and nodules develop, most commonly over the cheekbones after prolonged use of hydroquinone. Ironically, the patient usually has been using the hydroquinone to lighten the facial skin.

EPIDEMIOLOGY

The first reported cases of exogenous ochronosis were black women from South Africa who were using hydroquinone-containing bleaching creams at concentrations from 3.5% to 7.5% for 6 months or more.[1] As a result, in the early 1980s the cosmetic industry in South Africa was required to limit concentrations of the cream to 2%. Since then, the incidence of exogenous ochronosis in South Africa has remained high. In 1990, Weiss, Fabbro, and Kolisang[2] found an incidence of 31% of exogenous ochronosis in a gynecology outpatient department, and Hardwick et al[3] found in 1989 that 42% of his female patients were affected. Men may occasionally be affected as well.

Only 14 cases of exogenous ochronosis have been reported in the American literature as of 1995. This small figure stands in stark contrast to the millions of users of hydroquinone-containing products.

Black woman from the United States have been reported to have this condition, but the numbers for the United States are quite small. Grimes[4] points out that only 14 cases of exogenous ochronosis have been reported in the American literature as of 1995, and this small figure stands in stark contrast to the millions of users of hydroquinone-containing products. Most of these cases resulted from use of the 1% to 2% hydroquinone.

ETIOLOGY

The pathogenesis of ochronosis is not clear. The main contributory factors are the use of hydroquinone-containing creams and chronic sun exposure. The fibroblast seems intimately involved as well. The actual content and origin of the ochronotic fibers is still subject to debate. Findley, Morrison, and Simon[1] postulate that hydroquinone and other phenol compounds are able to alter elastin to form the ochronotic fibers and collagen to form the colloid milia. They note that the ochronotic fibers in the deeper dermis merge with ordinary elastotic fibers. This change could either occur via fibroblast uptake of the hydroquinone and subsequent disruption of production of elastin and collagen or via alteration of extracellular elastin and/or collagen. Hoshaw, Zimmerman, and Menter[5] agree with the premise that the ochronotic fibers are more closely related to elastin than to collagen based on their ultrastructural studies. In contrast, Phillips, Isaacson, and Carman[6] believe that the ochronotic fibers result from a breakdown of normal collagen. Penneys[7] has proposed that topically applied hydroquinone inhibits the activity of homogentisic acid oxidase in the skin, resulting in the local accumulation of homogentisic acid, which then polymerizes to form ochronotic pigment.

If and how the melanocyte plays a role in any of this is unclear. A potential lead in this area stems from a report by Hull and Procter.[8] They described a patient who suffered from both ochronosis and vitiligo (Figures 17-1 to 17-3), and noted that the ochronosis seemed to spare the areas of vitiligo. This suggests that perhaps the melanocyte plays a more important role in the formation of onchronosis than previously thought.

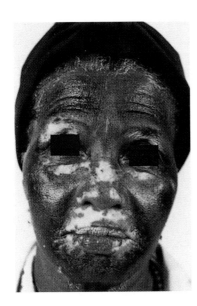

Figure 17-1   Distribution of exogenous ochronosis and vitiligo. (From Hull PR, Procter PR: *J Am Acad Dermatol* 22:529, 1990.)

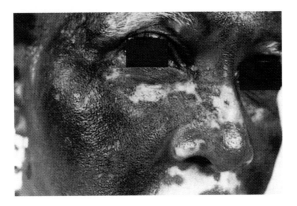

Figure 17-2   Ochronosis-sparing areas of vitiligo. (From Hull PR, Procter PR: *J Am Acad Dermatol* 22:529, 1990.)

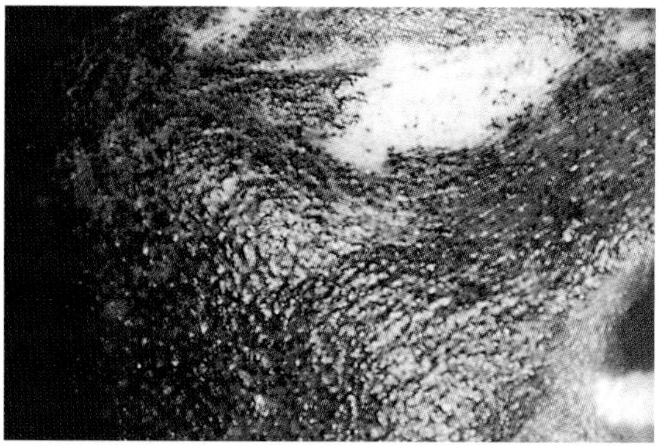

Figure 17-3   Coarse ochronotic textural changes and only scanty pigmented papules in area of vitiligo. (From Hull PR, Procter PR: *J Am Acad Dermatol* 22:529, 1990.)

Of note, hydroquinone is a phenolic compound like homogentisic acid. Other compounds have been reported to cause exogenous ochronosis (e.g., phenol-containing dressings for chronic wounds). It is unknown why whites are not affected, despite the large number of them using bleaching creams for melasma and other conditions.

Endogenous ochronosis is a totally separate disease that results from an autosomal recessively inherited deficiency in homogentisic acid oxidase. It leads to a buildup of oxidized homogentisic acid that is insoluble. Blue-black cartilage, most visible through the thin skin of the ears, is the result. The histologic changes of exogenous and endogenous ochronosis are virtually identical.

CLINICAL

The typical patient with exogenous ochronosis is a black woman who has been using a hydroquinone-containing bleaching cream on her face. She may experience initial skin lightening, but then the area begins to darken. She may change from one bleaching cream to another, trying to find one that reverses the effect. The initial clinical appearance is that of faint, macular, sooty pigmentation in the malar distribution. It may be reticulated or ripplelike. The sun-exposed bony prominences are preferred and include the forehead, temples, nose, and lower jaw. Presumably these are the areas where the cream is rubbed in most effectively. If allowed to progress, the skin may become indurated and studded with discrete, 1- to 2-mm, yellow-brown papules or glistening, jet-black, caviar-like papules. Keloidlike nodules and plaques may be seen in advanced cases. When examining the patient, both the barely visible sooty specks and the caviar-like nodules are best seen when the skin is stretched. Most of the sun-exposed skin may be affected in severe cases, including the sides and back of the neck, upper chest and back, and the extensor surfaces of the extremities. The creases around the eyes or the cavity of the pinna may be preferentially affected, presumably because night creams could be trapped there. A blue tint may be seen in the cavity of the auricle.

The typical patient with exogenous ochronosis is a black woman who has been using a hydroquinone-containing bleaching cream on her face. She may experience initial skin lightening, but then the area begins to darken.

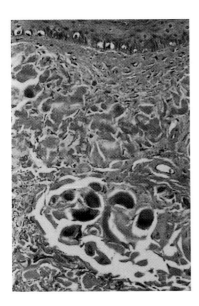

Figure 17-4   Ochronotic changes in pigmented skin. (From Hull PR, Procter PR: *J Am Acad Dermatol* 22:529, 1990.)

Coexistent ochronosis and allergic contact dermatitis to hydroquinone have been documented in one patient.[9]

HISTOLOGY

Histologically, one sees banana-shaped, yellow-brown globules of pigment in the papillary dermis (Figure 17-4). The lesions tend to be biggest and darkest just below the epidermis. Deeper, the fibers are more narrow and more yellow or green. A variable cellular infiltrate composed of lymphocytes, macrophages, epithelioid cells, and/or giant cells may be seen. Well-formed granulomas[10] and transepidermal elimination[11] have been reported. Jacyk[12] reported three patients with annular granulomatous lesions and systemic sarcoidosis. He concluded that annular granulomatous lesions in patients with exogenous ochronosis are a form of sarcoidosis.

When present and fully developed, the colloid milia are similar to the conventional colloid milia—eosinophilic, cracked, amorphous material devoid of ochronotic material. In intermediate phases of formation, the colloid milia might contain ochronotic material, usually in the diffuse form and seldom in the rod-shaped or banana form.[1] If the ear cartilage has been affected, ochronosis with fibrillar degeneration and chondrocytes filled with granules are seen in the outer third of the cartilage.[1]

As noted, the interpretation of ultrastructural studies has differed as to the possible origin of the ochronotic fibers. Hoshaw, Zimmerman, and Menter[5] have described them as "giant abnormal fibers that may be best termed *elastotic material.*" In contrast, others have concluded that the ochronotic fibers resemble collagen.[6]

TREATMENT

The hydroquinone should be discontinued and sunscreen used daily. Some have also prescribed hydrocortisone. The skin changes are often permanent, although some patients experience either significant lightening or shrinkage of the papular component. If papular lesions are prominent, surgical excision may be helpful.

REFERENCES

1. Findley GH, Morrison JGL, Simon IW: Exogenous ochronosis and pigmented colloid milium from hydroquinone bleaching creams, *Br J Dermatol* 93:613-622, 1975.
2. Weiss RM, Fabbro E, Kolisang P: Cosmetic ochronosis caused by bleaching creams containing 2% hydroquinone, *S Afr Med J* 77:373, 1990.
3. Hardwick N et al: Exogenous ochronosis: an epidemiological study, *Brit J Dermatol* 120:229-238, 1989.
4. Grimes PE: Melasma: etiologic and therapeutic considerations, *Arch Dermatol* 131:1453-1457, 1995.
5. Hoshaw RA, Zimmerman KG, Menter A: Ochronosislike pigmentation from hydroquinone bleaching creams in American blacks, *Arch Dermatol* 1221:105-108, 1985.
6. Phillips JI, Isaacson C, Carman H: Ochronosis in black south Africans who used skin lighteners, *Am J Dermatopath* 8:14-21, 1986.
7. Penneys NS: Ochronosislike pigmentation from hydroquinone bleaching creams, *Arch Dermatol* 121:1239-1240, 1985.
8. Hull PR, Procter PR: The melanocyte: an essential link in hydroquinone-induced ochronosis, *J Am Acad Dermatol* 22:529-531, 1990.
9. Camarasa JG, Serra-Baldrich E: Exogenous ochronosis with allergic contact dermatitis from hydroquinone: *Contact Dermatitis* 31:57-58, 1994.
10. Dogliotti M, Leibowitz M: Granulomatous ochronosis—a cosmetic-induced skin disorder in blacks, *S Afr Med J* 56:757-760, 1979.
11. Jordaan H, Van Niekerk DJT: Transepidermal elimination in exogenous ochronosis: a report of two cases, *Am J Dermatopathol* 18:1207-1211, 1991.
12. Jacyk WK: Annular granulomatous lesions in exogenous ochronosis are manifestation of sarcoidosis: *Am J Dermatopath* 17:18-22, 1995.

Chapter 18

Ainhum

Gary M. White

A inhum is a benign but disfiguring autoamputation of the fifth toe. It primarily affects east African men who walk barefoot. The term *ainhum* is derived from the word in the East African language of Nagos meaning "to saw."

ETIOLOGY

Chronic rotational stresses and trauma from walking barefoot are etiologic factors associated with ainhum. Common to most patients is a history of shoelessness for some years before onset of the disease. Decreased vascular supply may also play an etiologic role. Normally, the foot's blood is supplied by two intercommunicating arches, one each from the posterior and anterior tibial arches. Dent et al[1] reported an absence of the plantar arch and arterial branches (off the posterior tibial artery) in four of five patients. It remains unclear whether this is a congenital anomaly or results from an acquired vasculopathy. It has been theorized that the increased fibroblastic response to minor trauma in blacks in blacks is contributory, but keloids are not part of the clinical or histologic appearance.

The term ainhum *is derived from the word in the East African language of Nagos meaning "to saw." Common to most patients is a history of shoelessness for some years before onset of the disease.*

EPIDEMIOLOGY

Both men and woman are affected by ainhum, with a slight male predominance in most studies. Onset may be from age 7 to 75. Incidence varies tremendously based on the population studied. The disease is rare in the United States, but common in Africa. Cases have been reported in Brazil, Canada, the United States, Great Britain, Central and South America, Asia, and the former Soviet republics.

CLINICAL

Initially, a sulcus appears at the plantar junction of the fifth toe with the sole. It usually starts medially, coinciding with the plantar-digital fold, but it can occasionally occur beyond it. The groove then spreads around the toe until it forms a complete circle (Figure 18-1). Over time, the groove deepens until it ulcerates. Sterile bone re-

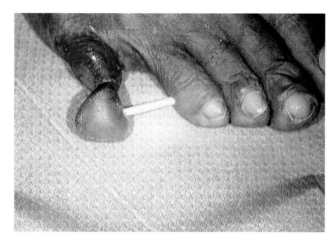

Figure 18-1 Ainhum with grade III severity. Autoamputation may occur shortly.

Table 18-1 Severity of Ainhum

Grade	Description
I	A groove only
II	Ulceration of the floor of the groove
III	Involvement of bone
IV	Autoamputation has occurred

From Cole GJ: *J bone Joint Surg* 47-B:43, 1965.

sorption then begins. The bone becomes spongy, and the soft tissue converts to an avascular fibrous cord. Ultimately, the toe may hang from the foot by a thin band of soft tissue. Spontaneous amputation can then occur. The majority of patients have both fifth toes affected, but unilateral involvement is also common; occasionally, the fourth toe may be affected. Cole and Ekwendeni[2] have graded the severity of the disease (Table 18-1).

Progression through the various stages may be rapid, progressing to autoamputation within a year, or it may be slow, arresting in grade I. In Cole and Ekwendeni's study, the average time to autoamputation was 5 years. Pain is common and is usually felt at the groove but at times may be felt distally. When the proximal phalanx fractures, severe pain and limping may result. Chronic maceration and infection of the groove is common and may give rise to edema of the dorsal aspect of the foot adjacent to the attachment of the toe.

HISTOLOGY

On low-power microscopic examination, a V-shaped depression is seen at the site of the groove. The epidermis exhibits moderate or severe hyperkeratosis with variable parakeratosis. Dermal inflammation is variable and may be composed of lymphocytes, plasma cells, and the occasional neutrophil or giant cell. The blood vessels are usually normal, but their lumens may be narrowed with intimal proliferation. The amount of subcutaneous tissue is reduced, and in some cases the dermis abuts the periosteum of the distal phalanx. Sterile absorption of bone occurs; in advanced cases, no bone is present at the groove site.

DIFFERENTIAL DIAGNOSIS

The differential diagnosis should include *pseudoainhum*, a term used to describe circumferential constriction of a digit (finger or toe). This condition resembles ainhum but is caused by a variety of disorders, including many of the keratodermas, leprosy, erythropoetic protoporphyria, Olmsted's syndrome, porokeratosis of Mibelli, and strangulation by hair or string.

TREATMENT

Trauma should be avoided, and the wearing of shoes or sandals is important. Amputation for a dangling digit may be necessary, although allowing autoamputation to occur is not unreasonable. Excision of the groove, followed by surgical Z-plasty, may be performed for all grade I lesions and early grade II lesions.[2] Any bacterial or fungal infection of the sulcus should be treated. Four cases of ainhum complicated by *Trichosporum* infection showed marked improvement with topical antifungal therapy.[3]

REFERENCES

1. Dent DM et al: Ainhum and angiodysplasia, *Lancet* 2:396, 1981.
2. Cole GJ, Ekwendeni M: Ainhum: an account of fifty-four patients with special reference to etiology and treatment, *J Bone Joint Surg Br* 47:43-51, 1965.
3. Kamalam A, Thambia AS: Ainhum, trichosporosis and Z-plasty, *Dermatologica* 162:372, 1981.

Chapter 19

Additional Skin Diseases

Gary M. White

PERIUMBILICAL PERFORATING PSEUDOXANTHOMA ELASTICUM

Perforating pseudoxanthoma elasticum is a rare, benign change of the skin about the umbilicus (Figure 19-1) and is most commonly seen in obese, multiparous, black or Mediterranean women.[1] White women may also be affected. The histologic appearance is similar to pseudoxanthoma elasticum (PXE), but systemic features of PXE are not found. The presumed etiologic process is the degeneration of middermal elastic fibers that then calcify and are finally extruded. The periumbilical area is thought to be important because the skin there is subject to much intermittent stretching after multiple pregnancies. Why darker-skinned patients are preferentially affected is unknown. Other names for this disease have been used, including *perforating calcific elastosis.*

The patient typically presents with a slowly enlarging, hyperpigmented, keratotic, periumbilical plaque. The central area is often flat, and the border is serpiginous. Some patients present with a background of yellow, cobblestone papules and nodules, with a few hyperkeratotic lesions.

Histologic examination shows short, gnarled, basophilic elastic fibers that stain positive for calcium. Transepidermal elimination of these altered fibers may be seen, which clinically gives rise to the hyperkeratotis or verrucous areas. The epidermis is usually acanthotic and may show pseudoepitheliomatous hyperplasia.

Classic PXE shold be excluded with an eye examination (angioid streaks) and a review of systems to include cardiac problems, hypertension, and gastrointestinal bleeding. Although there is no specific treatment, patients may be reassured that the condition is benign.

INHERITED PATTERNED LENTIGINOSIS IN BLACKS

The patient with inherited patterned lentiginosis has a striking involvement of the central face (Figure 19-2, *A, B*) and lips (Figure 19-2, *C*), with many small, discrete lentigos.[2] The dorsal hands and feet, buttocks, and elbows (Figure 19-2, *D*) may also be affected. Onset is in infancy or early childhood. There is no mucous membrane or internal involvement. Inheritance is autosomal dominant.

No treatment is usually needed. Laser therapy (e.g., with the 510-nm dye laser) may be used.[3]

210

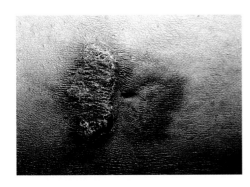

Figure 19-1 Hyperpigmented periumbilical plaque. (From Pruzan D, Rabbin PE, Heilman ER: *J Am Acad Dermatol* 26:642, 1992.)

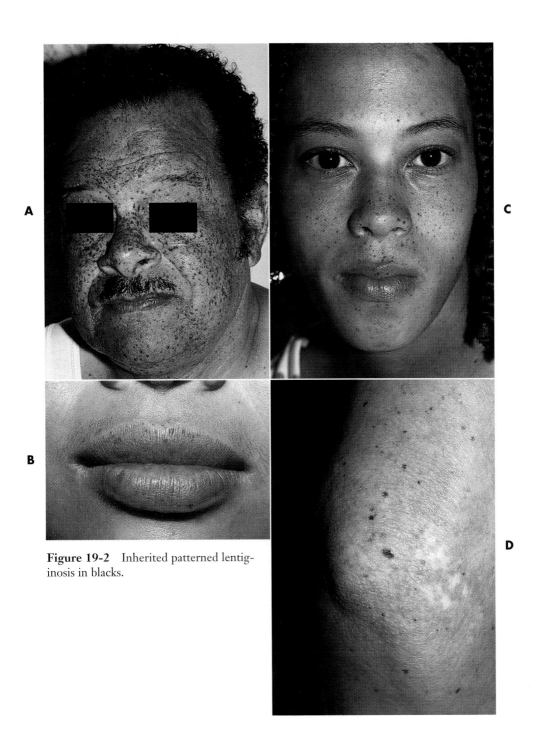

Figure 19-2 Inherited patterned lentiginosis in blacks.

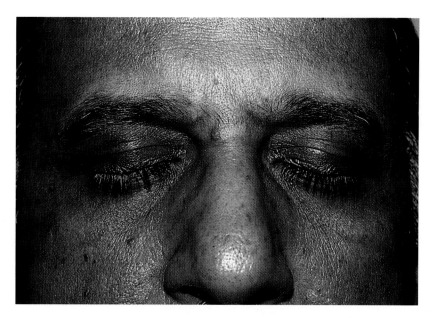

Figure 19-3   Familial periorbital melanosis in a man from India.

FAMILIAL PERIORBITAL MELANOSIS

The periorbital area is more darkly pigmented than the surrounding skin in inherited familial periorbital melanosis, an autosomal dominant disorder. Darker-skinned patients and those of Mediterranean descent are most commonly affected (Figure 19-3). Onset is in adolescence; the lower lid is usually involved first, followed by progression to the upper eyelid. Some fluctuation in the darkness of pigmentation may occur over time. Histologic studies show increased melanin granules in the basal and lower malpighian layers as well as the presence of many melanophages in the upper third of the dermis.[4] Clinically, however, no inflammation is seen. This disease should be distinguished from the pigmentation that may develop with a chronic dermatitis, such as atopic dermatitis.

PHOTODAMAGED ASIAN SKIN

The classic signs of photodamage—wrinkling, mottled pigmentation, actinic keratoses, a yellowish hue, solar elastosis, and lentigos—are easily recognized in the fair-skinned patient. More subtle changes that characterize photodamage in the Asian patient are less well appreciated.

Clinical

Pigmentary alterations are the main consequence to Asian skin of chronic UV exposure (Figure 19-4). Hyperpigmentation in the form of solar lentigos and melasma are common. Guttate hypomelanotic lesions also occur. It should be noted that melasma-like changes are seen in men as well as women. Both coarse and fine wrinkling may be seen but not to the extent that appears in skin types I and II.

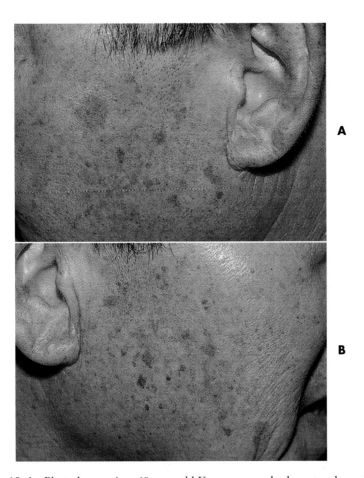

Figure 19-4   Photodamage in a 60-year-old Korean man who loves to play golf.

Treatment

The standard approach to treating photodamage is applicable here. Sun protection in the form of daily applicaton of sunscreen, sun avoidance, and the wearing of a hat is the basis for any treatment regimen. Tretinoin applied at bedtime is a helpful adjunct for both the pigmentary changes and the wrinkling.[5] Bleaching creams such as hydroquinone 3% to 4% applied twice daily or azelaic acid may be employed to lighten hyperpigmented areas. Chemical peels have also been used.

REFERENCES

1. Pruzan D, Rabbin PE, Heilman E: Periumbilical pseudoxanthoma elasticum, *J Am Acad Dermatol* 26:642-644, 1992.
2. O'Neill JF, James WD: Inherited patterned lentiginosis in blacks, *Arch Dermatol* 125:1231-1235, 1989.
3. Grekin RC et al: 510-nm pigmented lesion dye laser, *J Dermatol Surg Oncol* 19:380-387a, 1993.
4. Goodman RM, Belcher RW: Periorbital hyperpigmentation: an overlooked genetic disorder of pigmentation, *Arch Dermatol* 100:169-174, 1969.
5. Goh SH: The treatment of visible signs of senescence: the Asian experience, *Br J Dermatol* (suppl 35) 122:105-109, 1990.

Scalp and Hair Disease in the Black Patient

Amy J. McMichael

To recognize and treat pathologic conditions of the hair and scalp in black patients, it is first important to understand the normal state of the hair and scalp in this population. In any population there is a significant range of hair types and hair-care practices that makes generalizing impossible. The goal of the dermatologist must be to become familiar with the possible hair-care practices that may be encountered and be able to perform an appropriate, problem-directed history and physical examination.

Hair care for blacks is a billion dollar business that shows no signs of decline.[1,2] Black women, in particular, spend considerable time and money to achieve hairstyles mandated by current fashion trends, African heritage, societal demands, and/or personal expression. Two of the most important dilemmas many women of color face include choosing healthy hair-care regimens for coarse, wavy, and frizzy hair and avoiding hair-care practices that may have the potential to cause irreparable damage to the hair shaft and scalp. The key to providing acceptable medical advice for many of the hair disorders that occur in blacks lies in helping each patient address these issues in a way that still allows for personal expression and styling ease. This chapter will explore hair structure, styling agents, scalp and hair disease, and treatment regimens.

HAIR STRUCTURE

Scalp hair has long been a factor in the classification of the races.[3] For years, anthropologic classification systems of the hair have been described, none of which completely encompass the variety found in the black population. What can be observed are visible differences in the hair structure of people of different ethnic origins. Blacks often have clinically frizzier, woolier, or curlier hair compared with whites and Asians. These differences can make the hair in blacks more brittle and thus more sensitive to excessive manipulation. The physician who does not recognize these differences may recommend treatment for hair and scalp disease that is ineffective or that causes further damage to the already delicate hair shaft.

The black patient's hair shaft tends to be elliptical or flattened in cross section and spiral or tightly curled in its tertiary structure. Hair-shaft structure in the Asian patient tends to be round in cross section and relatively large in diameter.

The black patient's hair shaft tends to be elliptical or flattened in cross section and spiral or tightly curled in its tertiary structure. Hair-shaft structure in the Asian patient tends to be round in cross section and relatively large in diameter. The white patient's hair shaft usually has a structure that is somewhere between that of Asian and black patients. The hair shaft is round or oval in cross section, with a tertiary structure that varies from straight to wavy to helical.[4] Within each race, significant variations are seen as well. In blacks, the curled hair does not emanate from a straight follicle. Instead, the follicle where the hair is formed is just as curved as the hair itself.[5] Biochemical hair structures from different racial populations have been compared using various techniques, and no biochemical differences have as yet been elucidated.[6]

THE BASICS OF HAIR CARE

Hair-care practices are different for different ethnic groups. In the case of blacks, many hair-care products have been developed to meet the needs of this population. For many years, lubricating materials have been used to supplement the natural oils of the scalp. These products help to provide natural-looking, healthy hair; protection from the elements; and easy grooming. Straightening the curl of the hair has developed into a science of its own based on thermal and chemical methods. It is important to have an understanding of how these practices and products are used in grooming, so that a radically foreign procedure is not recommended by the dermatologist when scalp and hair treatment is needed. Not only will the patient often disregard therapy that is incompatible with usual practice as impossible to perform, but he or she may also lose faith in ever obtaining helpful medical advice.

Emollients for the hair are very commonly used to prevent flaking of the scalp and to add manageability to the hair.

Hair Care Products

Emollients

Emollients for the hair are very commonly used to prevent flaking of the scalp and to add manageability to the hair. They are most easily separated for discussion into two groups: liquid and solid preparations. Some authors choose to separate emollients by more specific characteristics of the product, such as pomades, oils, and brilliantines.[7] No matter which classification system is utilized, chemicals are used to produce a conditioning effect on the hair. For years, solid emollients (pomades are one form) have been used on virgin (untreated with heat or chemicals) curly or kinky hair[8] to allow for sheen in natural styles or to permit ease during braiding of hair. These products have also been used successfully as coating agents during heat-processing of curly hair and as finishing aids on chemically relaxed hair.[9] Patients will often refer to this kind of product as "hair grease." These thick products usually contain various mixtures of petrolatum, lanolin, and vegetable, mineral, or animal oils.[7,9,10] Thicker products are stiffened by the addition of waxes that also impart opacity to the various styling agents. Resins may also be added to increase the hair-grooming effectiveness of the formulation.[10] There is little to no water in these mixtures, which makes them reliable as protective agents against the elements,[10] but often messy to apply. For blacks who want a more sculptured hairstyle with little movement, these are ideal products. These products are usually packaged in jars or tubes to accommodate their ointment or creamy nature.

With the advent of chemical relaxing, many black women have decreased their use of thick hair emollients and increased their use of liquid emollients or moisturizers.[11] Thick lubricants are not usually necessary to protect hair from the elements when the hair is chemically relaxed. Oils (mineral and vegetable) are the primary lubricating agents in the liquid emollients, but liquid lanolin, which has good oil solubility, is sometimes added. These products are most often clear and homogenous,[10] presumably because they are more visually appealing. Coupling agents, such as acetylated glycerides, acetylated lanolin derivatives, and/or fatty esters, are used in these products to form solutions from usually immiscible chemicals.[10]

Liquid moisturizing agents containing oils mixed with silicone derivatives are among the newest hair moisturizers on the market. Many patients with chemically relaxed hair prefer these products over the thicker emollients because of the natural shine and lubrication they provide without greasiness.[11] Patients who desire a moisturizer but wish to maintain a bouncy look to the hair often prefer the silicone-derivative moisturizers. Some forms of this product are applied to freshly washed hair while the hair is still wet. Then the hair is styled as usual. Other forms of the volatile silicones are applied as finishing agents to styled hair to promote shine and reduce conditioner buildup between shampooings.

Other moisturizing liquid emollients include glycerin-based products that are sometimes referred to as *curl activators*. These products have been formulated for use on hair that is treated with a chemical curling agent, although it is sometimes used on virgin hair. Chemically relaxed and heat-straightened hair can benefit from treatment with glycerin-based products if they are washed out before styling. The glycerin does not repel moisture as well as other emollients and can cause reversion to the natural curl pattern,[9] limiting its usefulness.

Pitfalls of thick emollient use

Problems can arise from the use of thick hair emollients. Often these products are used to reduce scalp flaking by applying the ointment or cream diffusely and directly onto the scalp. This practice can make flaking less noticeable, but lanolin and some vegetable oil additives in thick products have been reported to worsen seborrheic dermatitis.[7] These products can also induce or worsen acne secondary to the comedogenic potential of lanolins and isopropyl myristate additives.[12-14] In the case of worsening acne or seborrheic dermatitis, any offending agent must be stopped, and mineral oil products can be substituted. For patients with fine hair, the greasy nature of these products can make the hair limp and difficult to curl. For these reasons, more liquid agents have been formulated to incorporate excellent coating properties without greasiness and to minimize follicular occlusion. Helpful recommendations to patients with acne secondary to emollient use are to wash their pillowcases frequently, wear clean scarves on their hair each night to protect their faces, or minimize use of the product on the scalp and hair.

Styling gel or spritz

Styling gels contain water, carbomer 940, and hydrolyzed animal protein, whereas the spritzes contain a copolymer of polyvinyl-pyrrolidine and vinyl acetate.[1,7] Both of these products are designed to form a thick, protective coating that dries on the hair and becomes very sticky to the touch. A very popular hairstyle among some black women is a style in which chemically relaxed or heat-straightened hair is moisturized, then treated with a styling gel, spritz, or both, and crafted into a sculptured hairstyle. Sculptured hairstyles are usually kept in place for 1 to 2 weeks before the hair is washed and restyled. Some patients prefer this style because there is relatively little upkeep needed between washings, and the surface of the hair is protected from the elements by the gel coating. Problems with this style include the drying effect these products have on the hair and potential worsening of seborrheic dermatitis from lanolin additives.[7]

Patients may often be tempted to leave this hairstyle intact for longer than 1 week to decrease upkeep further. Patients should be encouraged to wash these products out regularly to ensure healthy sloughing of scalp skin and to minimize drying of the hair shafts. If the hair is manipulated before the product is washed out, significant hair breakage can occur because the hair often becomes dry and brittle with the use of the product. These products are best used on healthy hair and/or saved for intermittent use to minimize hair damage.

Shampoo and conditioners

Most manufacturers have known for years that excessively curly hair can be damaged by shampoos that are not formulated properly for hair type. Shampoos for excessively curly hair should contain mild detergents, detangling chemicals, and a pH-balanced range of 4.5 to 5.5[1] to avoid combing damage and dry hair shafts. Since sebum secretions do not travel down and coat the hair shaft of curly and kinky hair as readily as straight hair, most black women need only wash their hair once to twice weekly. Patients who use coating products on the hair, such as spritz or gel, should be encouraged to wash at least weekly to minimize buildup of the product that will in turn require harsher shampoos.

The content and function of conditioners varies widely. Generally, excessively curly hair requires deeper conditioning than naturally straight hair. Since so many black women use a mixture of chemical relaxers and some form of heat in styling their hair, deep-penetrating conditioners are needed to coat the damaged cuticle.

Hair Restructuring Techniques

The above products treat the outer surface of the hair, but do not alter its underlying structure. Although many blacks choose natural curly or braided hairstyles, others prefer to straighten the hair for increased manageability, more styling options, or simply for personal preference. The following agents and procedures alter the structure of the hair, either temporarily or permanently.

Hot combing

The hot-combing process, also known as *pressing the hair*, works as a temporary method of straightening kinky or curly hair. In the early 1900s, Madame C. J. Walker received a patent for pioneering the use of a heated metal comb to smooth and soften curly hair.[15,16] With this technique, a metal comb is heated to high temperatures (150° to 500° Fahrenheit) by a heat source such as a small electric warmer, gas burner, or hot flame. Washed and dried hair is treated with an ointment-based lubricant, and the hot comb is slowly pulled through small sections of hair (Box 20-1). This process tem-

---

Box 20-1   Typical Hair Care Regimen for Hot-Combed Hair

Hair should be trimmed every 8 weeks.
Wash with moisturizing shampoo and condition with deep penetrating conditioner every week.
Liquid or thick emollient is applied to hair shafts and combed out to detangle.
The hot comb is heated and the hair is divided into small sections. The hot comb is run through one section at a time from the base of scalp to the ends of hair.
A curling iron is used to add body and curl.
Hair may be rolled loosely on curlers nightly to keep style.

porarily rearranges hydrogen and disulfide bonds within the hair shaft.[4,16,17] The hair remains straight until it is exposed to moisture. After straightening, the hair is usually curled with a curling iron for style. On rewetting, all signs of the hot-combing effect are lost, and the hair reverts to its original state.

Damage and approach to treatment

In recent years, the hot-comb method of thermal straightening of the hair has fallen out of favor with many black women because of the temporary nature of the process, the introduction of safe chemical relaxers, and the problems associated with the hot-combing procedure. Common problems include burning of the skin around the scalp that is accidently contacted by the hot comb[18] and overheating of the hair shaft, causing weakening and breakage.[16,17] Long-term use of the hot comb can cause severe damage to the hair shaft if the technique is not performed correctly. Ways to avoid hair shaft damage include having a well-trained professional performed the procedure, keeping hot combing to a maximum of once weekly, hot-combing only clean and dry hair, and obtaining regular trimmings of split ends every 6 to 8 weeks. If damage does ensue, cutting the damaged part of the hair shaft should be recommended. Possible challenges include patient resistance to cutting the hair. Although patients may recognize that the hair is damaged, it is often psychologically difficult to cut remaining hair if prior loss has been great. A moisturizing shampoo and conditioner should be used weekly, and a hair-coating agent such as a thick emollient can be used to protect against further damage from heat. An alternative is to discontinue all forms of heat and chemical manipulation until the damaged portion of the hair shafts can be completely trimmed. Often, this option is undesirable to patients if they have never worn their hair naturally. It is up to the dermatologist to suggest a regimen that may include heat or chemicals, but in a safe fashion.

A scarring form of hair loss called *hot comb alopecia* was described by LoPresti, Papa, and Kligman in 1968.[19] It was surmised that the oils used to lubricate the hair during the hot-combing process become heated, which causes them to travel down the hair shaft onto the scalp, leading to permanent scarring alopecia that is most prominent over the vertex of the scalp. More recent data suggest there may be other etiologies for this observed scarring process (see Follicular Degeneration Syndrome, p. 226) because there is often poor correlation between this form of alopecia and hot-comb use.[20]

Chemical relaxers

As long ago as the early 1900s, chemical agents have been used to straighten kinky or curly hair. Some of the early chemicals used included lye, hog lard, and boiled eggs.[15] Known as gassing, conking, or processing, these crude forerunners of the modern relaxers were used mostly by men. In the 1960s, chemical straighteners became more refined and less damaging to the hair and scalp, and more women began to utilize these products. Chemical relaxers are now the most common method of hair straightening used by black women.

Most chemical relaxers used on the hair in blacks contain sodium, potassium, or guanine hydroxides, sulfites, or thioglycolates. All of these chemicals work to produce a straight appearance by affecting the cysteine disulfide bonds of the hair. The chemicals are applied first to virgin hair from the scalp to the ends of the hair shaft. The scalp is often coated with a protective agent such as petroleum jelly before application of the relaxer. The relaxer is kept on the hair for 15 to 20 minutes and then rinsed out completely. A neutralizing shampoo follows the rinsing step. After shampooing, the hair is either set on rollers and dried under a hood dryer or blown dry and curled with a curling iron. Some blacks (men and women) use chemical relaxers to loosen the curl of the hair and then wear the hair in a natural style. As the hair grows, the chemical relaxer is applied only to the new growth of hair, with special care not to overlap the chemical onto previously treated hair. The reapplication of chemical to new growth is usually performed every 6 to 12 weeks and can prevent texture differences that may cause breakage during grooming[18] (Box 20-2). There are different degrees of hair shaft resistance to chemical relaxing agents observed in the hair of blacks that do not appear to correspond to hair shaft thickness or tightness of wave pattern[21]; for instance, a patient with wavy hair may observe less straightening with a relaxer than someone with extremely curly, coarse hair.

Most chemical relaxers used on the hair in blacks contain sodium, potassium, or guanine hydroxides, sulfites, or thioglycolates. All of these chemicals work to produce a straight appearance by affecting the cysteine disulfide bonds of the hair.

Hydroxide relaxers usually come packaged in three strengths: mild, normal, and strong, to accommodate different resistances to the relaxer. Average percentages of sodium hydroxide in the various relaxer strengths are 1.85% to 2.0%, 2.06% to 2.2%, and 2.25% to 2.4%, respectively.[1] These relaxers work indirectly via the hydroxyl group of the chemical that forms a covalent and permanent bond between a carbon group and a sulfur atom of the cysteine in the hair, which in turn causes the formation of a reactive double bond between carbon groups.[15] This results in the formation of final products with stable covalent bonds, which cause permanent straightening of the hair. The sodium and potassium hydroxides are the strongest relaxers and allow for the most straightening of curly hair; however, they are also the most likely to cause scalp and hair damage.[18] Still, they remain the most commonly used form of relaxers.

Guanine hydroxide relaxers are typically packaged as calcium hydroxide with guanine carbonate in a separate container. The consumer or hair stylist adds the products together, which sparks a chemical reaction to produce guanine hydroxide, or the "no lye" relaxer. Once mixed, the product must be used immediately. These chemicals are frequently marketed for home use because they are typically less damaging to the hair and scalp than "lye" (sodium hydroxide) relaxers.[21]

Sulfites work through a different mechanism than hydroxide chemicals. The sulfite breaks the disulfide bonds of the hair to form sulfhydryl groups.[15] This mechanism of action forms less reactive end products than the hydroxide relaxers, so hair relaxation with sulfite relaxers tends to be less permanent. The reversion of the hair back to a natural wave pattern soon after application of the bisulfite chemicals has led to use of

---

Box 20-2   Typical Hair-Care Regimen for Relaxed Hair

Relaxer should be applied to new growth every 6 to 8 weeks.
Hair should be trimmed every 8 weeks.
Hair is washed 1 to 2 times weekly with moisturizing shampoo and conditioned with moisturizing conditioner.
A clear, silicone coating agent is applied to coat hair shafts.
Hair is blown dry or set on rollers under a hood dryer.
If blown dry, curling iron is used to curl hair, and hair may be loosely rolled on rollers nightly to keep style.
Application of a non–alcohol-containing hair spray for hold and/or thin emollient for shine and weather protection should be done daily.

this product on hair with a more Caucasoid texture.[7] These chemicals also require neutralization via alkalinizing agents. Sulfite relaxers are suitable for home use because their low reactivity also makes them less damaging to the hair than some other agents.[7]

The last form of chemical straightening agent is the thioglycolate agents. Technically, these agents relax the natural curl pattern of the hair and reset it in a curly or wavy pattern often referred to as a *chemical curl*, *Jheri curl*, or *S-curl*. Lately, the use of these chemicals has been less popular than the use of relaxing agents, partially because of the high upkeep required by this style and because of the severe hair damage that can occur. These chemicals are similar to those used in the permanent waving solutions used predominantly by whites. The thioglycolate reduces disulfide bonds, allowing reformation of the hair in the shape of the rods around which the hair is wound. This is usually a one- or two-step process consisting of one or two applications of ammonium thioglycolate in different concentrations ranging from 4% to 9.5%.[20,21] After 20 to 50 minutes, the chemical is washed out and a neutralizer such as sodium hydroxide is applied, which stops the thioglycolate process via oxidation and subsequent reformation of disulfide bonds. After the chemical curling procedure, a moisturizer containing glycerine and propylene glycol is used daily. The glycerine provide shine and the propylene glycol provides moisturization without buildup. A curl activator cream consisting of oils and humectants is also applied daily to activate the curls (make them bouncy and flexible) without weighing the hair down.[22] A comb-out spray containing silicone and lanolin is optimal for added sheen.

The thioglycolate reduces disulfide bonds, allowing reformation of the hair in the shape of the rods around which the hair is wound.

Damage and approach to treatment

Although chemical relaxers have revolutionized the hair care industry for black women, there are several problems that are constant reminders of how much work is still needed to decrease damaging side effects. The main problems associated with use of these products are hair shaft dryness, increased fragility of the hair cuticle (overporosity),[15,16] and the lesser problem of skin damage.[21] The physical examination of a patient with chemically damaged hair may show extensive broken hairs, diffuse baldness, and/or inflamed skin[17] (Figure 20-1). Light microscopy will often show a trichorrhexis nodosa pattern, which is thought to be an acquired weakness of the hair shaft caused by physical trauma.[23,24] In this disorder, small, beaded swellings are present along the hair shaft along with loss of cuticle. Scanning electron micrograph studies of healthy hair shafts after hydroxide chemical relaxing show cuticular abrasion and fusion,[15] both of which can lead to the observed fragility of the hair shaft. Moisturizing shampoos used immediately after chemical treatment can repair some of this overporosity.[15] In addition to the shaft becoming overporous, the elasticity of the hair can be severely decreased.[25] Measurements of tensile strength (elasticity) of hair that has been chemically relaxed by lye or no-lye chemicals shows an average loss of 19% to 40% of its strength.[21]

Other reported complications of relaxer use include a primary irritant contact dermatitis of the skin to relaxers[16] and fibrosis and inflammation of the scalp associated with alopecia.[26] Although there are significant data to support the cause and effect relationship between relaxer use and scarring alopecia, there is still a need for prospective or case-control evaluations of the nature of this relationship.

The damage that occurs with the thioglycolate chemicals is similar to that of the relaxing agents. Transmission electron microscopy (TEM) shows damage to the exocuti-

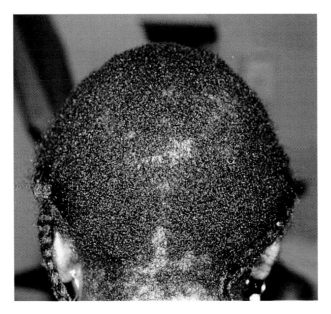

Figure 20-1 Note severe and uneven hair breakage in this patient secondary to acute chemical relaxer damage. The patient was reluctant to cut the two braids, which was the only hair spared from breakage.

Box 20-3 Repair Regimen for Damaged Relaxed Hair

Hair is trimmed at least every 8 weeks.
All damaged areas are cut until healthy hair shaft is visible.
Hair is washed with a moisturizing shampoo weekly.
Deep conditioner is used weekly to twice weekly.
A silicone coating agent should be used before drying hair.
Minimize use of blow dryer and curling iron (and other heat and traction
   sources).
No further chemicals should be used until hair is healthy.
A thin cream emollient should be used to coat hair after styling.
Hair spray and spritz use should be minimized.

---

cle of the thioglycolate-treated hair shaft, suggesting that not all of the disulfide bonds are reformed and that the treated hair is not as strong as before chemical processing.[15] TEM studies also show that over-neutralization can cause breakage of the reformed disulfide bonds, resulting in further damage. Overprocessing with the thioglycolate agents can lead to significant hair breakage because tensile strength loss can be as high as 56%.[21] The use of these agents can result in alopecia as described by Bulengo-Ransby,[27] who reported a case of verrucal alopecia occurring after thioglycolate use.

Overall, chemical relaxers are helpful grooming agents when used appropriately. It is important that patients with already damaged hair seek out professionals to apply relaxers if this is the preferred hair-care regimen. Using a thick substance, such as petroleum jelly, on the scalp during relaxer application may lessen relaxer-associated skin irritation. Also, maintaining a regimen of regular hair trims and keeping the relaxer applications to no closer than 6 weeks apart can make a large difference in the appearance of the hair shaft (Box 20-3).

HAIR AND SCALP DISORDERS

There are a number of hair and scalp disorders that occur more frequently among blacks than in other populations. A multifactorial etiology explains the severity of many of these disorders, with some hair-care practices worsening preexisting conditions.

Traction Alopecia

Many dermatologists are faced with children, usually female, and women who have experienced a symmetric loss or thinning of hair at the frontal and temporal hair line. This hair loss is commonly related to traction; it may be acute in onset, but is usually a chronic complaint. Referred to as *traction alopecia* and *traumatic alopecia marginalis*, this common form of alopecia can present as significant hair loss in any area of the scalp where tension has been put on the hair (Figure 20-2). Over the years, the literature has emphasized the traction component of this process rather than the traumatic elements that may also cause broken and damaged hair.[28,29] Though reported in women of many races, traction alopecia is frequently seen in the black population. The practices of tight braiding and hairstyles that require a straight appearance obtained with the use of drying agents, traction, and/or rubber bands often lead to this frontal hair loss. The mechanism of loss is thought to be a mechanical loosening of the hairs from the follicle accompanied by follicule-based inflammation.[17] Clinically, there may be accompanying folliculitis,[28] scattered broken hairs remaining, and prominent follicular hyperkeratosis[17] around follicles devoid of hair.

The practices of tight braiding and hairstyles that require a straight appearance obtained with the use of drying agents, traction, and/or rubber bands often lead to this frontal hair loss.

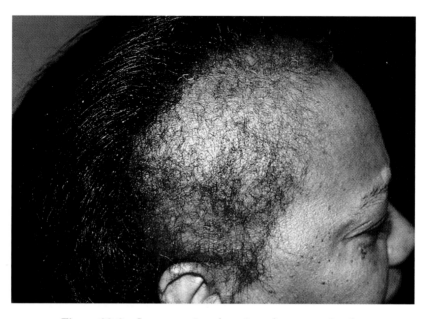

Figure 20-2   Severe traction alopecia at the temporal scalp.

Histologically, early traction alopecia can show scant perifollicular inflammation[30] with occasional follicle-based pustules. Biopsy from later-stage disease shows mild to moderate perifollicular inflammation, often with patchy loss of follicles and mild dermal fibrosis.[31]

Treatment

The mainstay of treatment for traction alopecia lies in correct diagnosis and discontinuing all practices that put tension on the hair. Early in the course of the disease, avoidance of manipulation of the hair in the affected areas is very successful in allowing regrowth. Often patients employ styling techniques that they may not consider to be traction-causing practices. Specific questioning of the patient should always be conducted regarding use of hair rollers,[32] stiff gels at the hair line, tight braids,[33] work-related head gear, and/or hair pieces attached with glue or tight stitches. If folliculitis is present, oral and/or topical antibiotics may be used. If hair loss is extensive and biopsy reveals significant inflammation, a trial of local low-dose intralesional steroid injections may help to decrease localized inflammation, thereby permitting hair growth.[31] Decreasing manipulation of the hair usually provides only limited improvement because there is often fibrosis in the place of follicular units. If the traction alopecia is long-standing, it may become permanent. In this case, punch graft and rotation flap hair transplantation have been successful treatments.[29] Advantages of a surgical treatment are the relatively low risk of major side effects and the relatively simple nature of the procedures. Disadvantages include the need for specialized surgical knowledge, the risk of prominent scarring from the procedure,[34] and the possibility of telogen effluvium causing temporary hair loss at the graft site.[35]

The mainstay of treatment for traction alopecia lies in correct diagnosis and discontinuing all practices that put tension on the hair.

Seborrheic Dermatitis

The wide geographic prevalence of seborrheic dermatitis is clear, but the role that racial variation plays is not clear.[4] As previously mentioned, there are reports of lanolin-containing products worsening this disease in some patients.[7] Seborrheic dermatitis may also be more noticeable in patients who wash their hair less than once weekly. To address the severity of seborrheic dermatitis effectively, it is imperative to find out the number of times per week the patients washes his or her hair, what hair styling products are used, and what previous antidandruff products have been tried.

Seborrheic dermatitis may also be more noticeable in patients who wash their hair less than once weekly.

One must be careful not to prescribe a regimen that includes washing the hair daily *with antidandruff shampoos or using a topical steroid in* solution *form.*

Treatment

When seborrheic dermatitis occurs in blacks, one must be careful not to prescribe a regimen that includes washing the hair daily with antidandruff shampoos or using a topical steroid in solution form. Although this may be an accepted approach to seborrheic dermatitis in some patients, this regimen would be unlikely to work well for most black patients. First, washing the hair daily is not a common practice among people who use chemical straighteners and heat for styling. Daily washings would be quite time-consuming and drying to the hair shaft, and could possibly cause damage. Next, solution-based products will often reverse the affects of thermal straightening and lead to difficulty in styling. Instead of steroid solutions, medium-potency steroid ointments or creams can be used daily at first and then be tapered to 2 to 3 times weekly as symptoms improve. An ointment containing 3% salicylic acid with 3% precipitated sulfur mixed in equal parts steroid and petrolatum can be useful to decrease scaling and pruritus.[17] Finally, the shampoos that are best for treatment of scaling dermatoses are often extremely harsh on excessively curly hair. A moisturizing conditioner either mixed with the anti-dandruff shampoo[16] or used after the shampoo will help to prevent brittle hair. Shampooing can be done once to twice weekly (Box 20-4). When a scaling scalp eruption begins in children, with or without accompanying hair loss, it is important to rule out tinea capitis before assuming the diagnosis is seborrheic dermatitis[36] (Figure 20-3).

Acne Keloidalis

For more information about acne keloidalis, see Chapter 9.

Box 20-4   Treatment Regimen for Seborrheic Dermatitis

Wash hair twice weekly for 1 month.
Alternate use of zinc-, tar-, ketaconazole-, and selenium sulfide–containing shampoos.
Follow medicated shampoos with usual shampoo to hair shafts only.
Midpotency topical steroid cream or ointment should be applied to the scalp daily for 1 week, then 3 to 4 times weekly.
Minimize use of nonmedicated products on the scalp.
Deep conditioner should be used on hair shafts only.
Follow usual hair-care regimen.

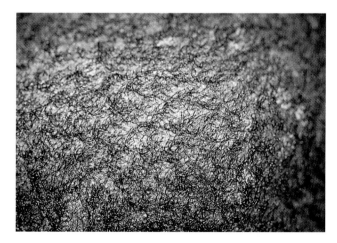

Figure 20-3   Tinea capitis in a child. The condition resembles seborrheic dermatitis.

Perifolliculitis Capitis Abscedens et Suffodiens

Perifolliculitis capitis abscedens et suffodiens, also known as *dissecting cellulitis*, is an uncommon chronic inflammatory disorder of the scalp. It occurs most commonly in black men, but can also be seen in women. It is characterized by large, tender, and fluctuant cysts and sinus tracts on the vertex and occipital scalp (Figures 20-4 and 20-5). Hair loss is often permanent in this disorder and is secondary to the severity and chronicity of scalp inflammation. Keloids may also form over the scalp in association with the active eruption. Histology reveals keratotic plugging of follicles with a dense, mixed-cell infiltrate involving the follicle and perifollicular dermis, often with extension to subcutaneous fat. The destructive infiltrate ultimately progresses to scar formation and fibrosis of the dermis. Pathogenesis of this disorder is unknown because skin samples taken from the affected site are usually sterile,[37] but follicular plugging via keratin with ensuing reactive granulomatous inflammation is thought to contribute to disease expression.[38] It is very important to exclude a persistant *Staphylococcus* infection, which

---

It is very important to exclude a persistant Staphylococcus *infection, which can be cleared with long-term antibiotics.*

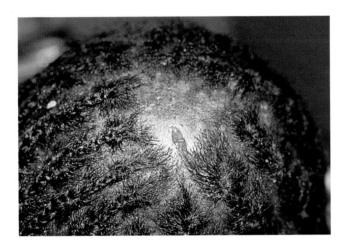

Figure 20-4   Active dissecting cellulitis with purulent drainage from a superficial sinus tract.

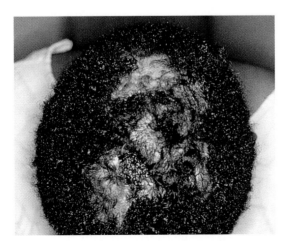

Figure 20-5   Chronic dissecting cellulitis with severe scarring, hair loss, and keloid formation.

can be cleared with long-term antibiotics. Repeated cultures should always be performed, and any positive cultures should be treated.

Treatment of dissecting cellulitis is often frustrating for the physician and the patient. Acute treatment regimens can include oral antibiotics, short courses of oral steroid tapers,[39] intralesional steroids, and incision and drainage of specific fluctuant nodules.[40] Other reported successful treatments include oral zinc therapy,[41] oral isotretinoin,[42] and wide local resection of the involved scalp followed by split-thickness grafting.[43] Treatment of the scalp with x-ray epilation has also been tried with success,[44] but several authors have questioned the use of x-ray treatment because there has been a report of de novo cancer in a patient at the site of dissecting cellulitis.[37] Often, the natural history of the cellulitis is dissipation after several years, but treatment should always be undertaken to avoid unnecessary suffering and scarring. Because treatment is often begun after significant scarring has already occurred, it may be necessary to discuss with the patient what to expect in terms of permanent scarring and/or hair loss.

Follicular Degeneration Syndrome

In recent years, the belief that hot combing the hair causes a scarring alopecia has been questioned. The prevalence of blacks using this method of hair straightening has declined sharply, seemingly without significant decline in the prevalence of the unexplained scarring alopecia that occurs on the vertex of the scalp in many black women. Clinically, these patients present between the ages of 22 and 80 with a marked loss of follicular openings and shiny skin over the vertex with notable hair loss that often extends to the frontal scalp (Figure 20-6). Past descriptions suggested that this disease was clinically similar and histologically indistinguishable from classic pseudopelade.[4] A retrospective analysis of 10 women thought to have hot-comb alopecia showed poor correlation of hot comb use with alopecia,[20] and these women were thought to have a newly described entity termed *follicular degeneration syndrome*. More recently, Sperling et al[45] have described this same clinical syndrome in black men.

In recent years, the belief that hot combing the hair causes a scarring alopecia has been questioned.

A common histologic link found in one report suggests these patients have premature desquamation of the inner root sheath,[20] though this commonality has not been found in a group of clinically similar patients.[31] Biopsy usually shows a decreased number of follicular units with fibrosis in the place of follicular units.[20] Varying levels of inflammation can often be seen, ranging from sparse to extreme perifollicular lymphohistiocytic infiltrates. Best seen on vertical sectioning, the biopsies will often show a coalescence of follicular units to form one unit with multiple hairs[46] (Figure 20-7). As mentioned previously, several authors have reported a scarring alopecia that has been temporally or historically related to chemical relaxers,[27] but it is not yet clear what role heredity, relaxing agents, and other hair-care practices may play in this very disfiguring hair loss syndrome seen in so many black women.

Treatment

Treating this form of scarring alopecia has been a challenge because pathogenesis is still not clear. For now, empiric treatments have been moderately successful in controlling symptoms and in slowing the progression of disease. Since no formal trials have been performed, it is not clear how much recovery will occur with any given treatment.

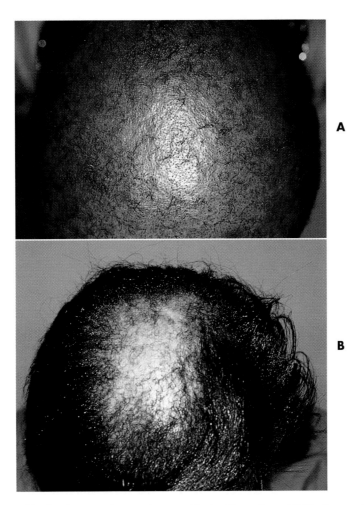

Figure 20-6   Follicular degeneration syndrome with significant loss of follicular openings and alopecia on frontal scalp and vertex.

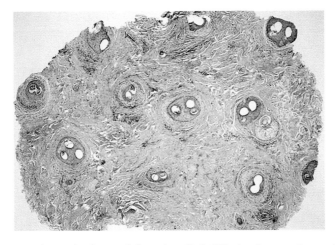

Figure 20-7   Histology of a form of alopecia called *follicular degeneration syndrome* showing fibrosis around follicles, with coalescence of follicles.

For symptoms of pruritus or tenderness, with or without histologic evidence of inflammation, oral antibiotics and topical steroid ointments have been used as antiinflammatory agents.[45] Extreme symptoms and significant histologic perifollicular infiltrates can be improved with local intralesional steroid injections monthly for 3 to 6 months.[17] Some authors have found antimalarials to be useful in treatment of this disease.[17]

Pseudofolliculitis Barbae

For more information about pseudofolliculitis barbae, see Chapter 12.

Psychosocial Effects of Hair Loss

Many of the aforementioned hair and scalp disorders cause temporary or permanent hair loss and/or disfigurement. Hair plays a major role in defining individuality and appearance. As a result, alopecia can negatively influence self-esteem and cause tremendous psychologic upheaval. Even when clinical disease is controlled, alopecia alone can cause depression and negatively influence quality of life.[47] It is important to address the clinical hair disorder as well as the emotional role hair loss may play. Most patients will cue the physician on what aspects of their hair disorder are most worrisome. It is imperative for the dermatologist to give patients this chance to air these concerns and help them deal with the emotional sequelea of hair disorders.

SUMMARY

Treating scalp and hair disorders is challenging because of the emotional nature of hair loss and because pathogenesis is lacking for so many hair disorders. Treating black patients can add an extra layer of complexity to this treatment if the dermatologist is not familiar with hair-care practices (Boxes 20-5 and 20-6). By no means are blacks a homogeneous population, and the treatments, products, and hair structures described here are, at best, generalizations. It takes an enlightened dermatologist to effectively treat hair disorders in patients of different ethnicities and hair-care practices. There will always remain a need to personalize treatment for each patient.

Box 20-5   Typical Hair-Care Regimen for Braided Hair

Hair is trimmed at least every 8 weeks.
Hair is washed and conditioned with moisturizing products every week or more frequently.
Hair is braided loosely at base of scalp with or without extensions added.
Braids should be removed and hair "rested" every 2 months.

Box 20-6   Typical Hair-Care Regimen for Natural Styles

Hair is trimmed at least every 8 weeks.
Hair is washed and conditioned with moisturizing products every week or more frequently.
Hair is coated with a liquid or thick emollient for protection and shine.

REFERENCES

1. Syed AN: Ethnic hair care: history, trends and formulation, *Cosmet Toil* 108:99-107, 1993.
2. Bonner LB: *Good Hair,* New York, 1990, Crown Trade Paperbacks.
3. Trotter M: Anthropometry: a review of the classification of hair, *Am J Phys Anthropol* 24:105-126, 1938.
4. Rook A, Dawber R: *Diseases of the hair and scalp,* Oxford, 1982, Blackwell Scientific Publications.
5. Lindelof B et al: Human hair form, *Arch Derm* 124:1359-1363, 1988.
6. Rook A: Racial and other genetic variations in hair form, *Br J Dermatol* 92:599-600, 1975.
7. Wilborn WS: Disorders in hair growth in African Americans. In Olsen EA, ed: *Disorders of hair growth,* New York, 1994, McGraw-Hill.
8. Corbett JF: The chemistry of hair care products, *J Soc Dyers and Colorists* 92:285-303, 1976.
9. Drealos ZD: Black individuals require special products for hair care, *Cosmet Dermatol* 6:19-20, 1993.
10. Goode ST: Hair pomades, *Cosmet Toil* 94:71-74, 1979.
11. Brooks G, Burmeister F: Black hair care ingredients, *Cosmet Toil* 103:93-96, 1988.
12. Kligman AM, Mills OH: Acne cosmetica, *Arch Dermatol* 106:843-850, 1972.
13. Plewig G, Fulton JE, Kligman Am: Pomade acne, *Arch Dermatol* 101:580-584, 1970.
14. Fulton JE, Pay SR, Fulton III JE: Comedogenicity of current therapeutic products, cosmetics, and ingredients in the rabbit ear, *J Am Acad Dermatol* 10:96-105, 1984.
15. Harris RT: Hair relaxing, *Cosmet Toil* 94:51-56, 1979.
16. Halder RM: Hair and scalp disorders in blacks, *Cutis* 32:378-380, 1983.
17. Scott DA: Disorders of the hair and scalp in blacks, *Dermatol Clin* 6:387-395, 1988.
18. Joyner M: Hair care in the black patient, *J Ped Health Care* 2:281-287, 1988.
19. LoPresti P, Papa CM, Kligman AM: Hot comb alopecia, *Arch Dermatol* 98:234-238, 1968.
20. Sperling LC: The follicular degeneration syndrome in black patients, *Arch Dermatol* 128:68-74, 1992.
21. Khalil EN: Cosmetic and hair treatments for the black consumer, *Cosmet Toil* 101:51-58, 1986.
22. Brooks GB, Lewis A: Treatment regimens for "styled" black hair, *Cosmet Toil* 98:59-68, 1983.
23. Whiting DA: Structural abnormalities of the hair shaft, *J Am Acad Dermatol* 16:1-25, 1987.
24. Price VH: Office diagnosis of structural hair anomalies, *Cutis* 15:231-240, 1975.
25. O'Donoghue MN: Hair cosmetics, *Dermatol Clinics* 5:619-626, 1987.
26. Nicholson AG et al: Chemically induced cosmetic alopecia, *Br J Dermatol* 128:537-541, 1993.
27. Bulengo-Ransby SM: Chemical and traumatic alopecia from thioglycolate in a black woman, *Cutis* 49:99-103, 1992.
28. Sleyan AH: Traction alopecia, *Arch Dermatol* 78:395-398, 1958.
29. Earles RM: Surgical correction of traumatic alopecia marginalis or traction alopecia in black women, *J Dermatol Surg Oncol,* 12:78-82, 1986.
30. Spencer GA: Alopecia luminaris frontalis, *Arch Dermatol Syphilol* 44:1082-1085, 1941.
31. McMichael AJ: Unpublished results.
32. Lipnik MJ: Traumatic alopecia from brush rollers, *Arch Dermatol* 84:183-185, 1961.
33. Rudolph RI, Klein AW, Decherd JW: Corn-row alopecia, *Arch Dermatol* (letter) 108:134, 1973.
34. Brown MD, Johnson T, Swanson N: Extensive keloids following hair transplantation, *J Dermatol Surg Oncol* 16:867-869, 1990.
35. Earles M: Hair transplantation, scalp reduction, and flap rotation in black men, *J Dermatol Surg Oncol* 12:87-96, 1986.
36. Brauner GJ: Cutaneous disease in black children, *Am J Dis Child* 137:488-496, 1983.
37. Williams CN et al: Dissecting cellulitis of the scalp, *Plast Reconstr Surg* 77:378-382, 1986.
38. Moyer DG: Perifolliculitis capitis abscedens et suffodiens, *Arch Dermatol* 85:580-584, 1962.
39. Adrian RM, Arndt KA: Perifolliculitis capitis: successful control with alternate day corticosteroids, *Ann Plast Surg* 4:166-169, 1980.
40. Kenney JA: Management of dermatoses peculiar to negroes, *Arch Dermatol* 91:126-129, 1965.

41. Berne B, Venge P, Ohman S: Perifolliculitis capitis abscedens et suffodiens (Hoffman), *Arch Dermatol* 121:1028-1030, 1985.

42. Schewach-Millet M, Ziv R, Shapira D: Perifolliculitis capitis abscedens et suffodiens treated with isotretinoin (letter), *J Am Acad Dermatol* 15:1291-1292, 1986.

43. Kantor GR, Ratz JL, Wheeland RG: Treatment of acne keloidalis nuchae with carbon dioxide laser, *J Am Acad Dermatol* 14:263-267, 1986.

44. McMullan FH, Zeligman I: Perifolliculitis capitis abscedens et suffodiens, *Arch Dermatol* 73:259, 1956.

45. Sperling LC et al: Follicular degeneration syndrome in men, *Arch Dermatol* 130:763-769, 1994.

46. White W: Personal communication, 1997.

47. van der Donk J et al: Quality of life and maladjustment associated with hair loss in women with alopecia androgentica, *Soc Sci Med* 33:159-163, 1994.

Dermal Melanocytic Lesions and Other Skin Conditions Common in the Asian Patient

Gary M. White

The pigmentation of nevomelanocytic nevi, lentigos, café au lait spots (CALS), etc., results from melanocytes in the epidermis. In contrast, dermal melanocytic lesions such as nevus of Ota, nevus of Ito, and Mongolian spots result from melanin-producing cells in the dermis. The blue color that characterizes these lesions results from the Tyndall effect (i.e., the scattering of the shorter wavelengths of light as it passes through the skin).

The blue color that characterizes these lesions results from the Tyndall effect (i.e., the scattering of the shorter wavelengths of light as it passes through the skin).

NEVUS OF OTA

Epidemiology

The nevus of Ota is a facial, dermal, melanocytic lesion common in the Asian patient. Onset is bimodal, with the larger peak at birth or soon after and the smaller peak at adolescence. Nearly all lesions appear by age 30. The incidence in the Japanese population has been estimated to be from 0.1% to 0.2%. Females predominate.

Clinical

The nevus of Ota is characterized by a unilateral, blue-black or brown pigmented patch in the distribution of the trigeminal nerve (predominately V1 and V2) (Figures 21-1 to 21-3). This usually corresponds to the forehead, temple, eyelid, nose, ear, and/or scalp. Pigmentation may also be found in the oral mucosa, sclera, or lympanic membrane. Ocular involvement may take the form of hyperpigmentation of the sclera, iris, conjunctiva, choroid, or optic disc. Rarely, ocular,[1] cutaneous, or intracranial melanoma may be associated.[2]

The nevus of Ota is characterized by a unilateral, blue-black or brown pigmented patch in the distribution of the trigeminal nerve (predominantly V1 and V2).

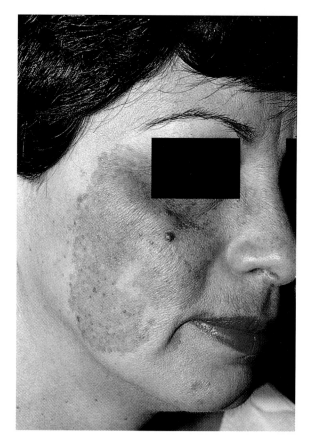

Figure 21-1   Nevus of Ota in an adult woman.

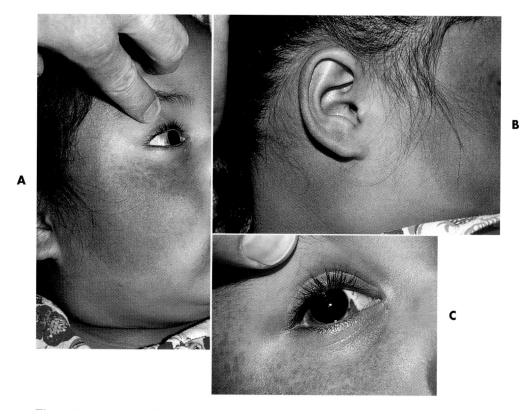

Figure 21-2   Nevus of Ota in a young girl **(A).** Note the extension to the ears and neck **(B)** and the scleral pigmentation **(C).**

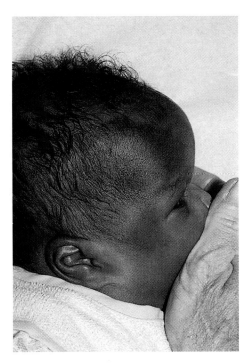

Figure 21-3   Nevus of Ota in a black child.

Treatment

The Q-switched ruby and the Nd:YAG lasers have been used effectively in the treatment of nevus of Ota.[3,4] Often, multiple treatments are needed.[5] Alternatively, skin abrasion followed after healing by cryotherapy using carbon dioxide snow has been used successfully.[6]

ACQUIRED BILATERAL NEVUS OF OTA-LIKE MACULES

Clinical

Blue-brown or slate gray macules distributed symmetrically on the cheeks, forehead, temples, eyelid, or nose is characteristic of acquired bilateral nevus of Ota-like macules (Figure 21-4). The patient is almost always an Asian or darkly pigmented woman. In a series of 320 patients, no men were found.[7] In most cases, the disease presents after 20 years of age.[8,9] The lesions are bilateral in contrast to the most common presentation of nevus of Ota. When the nevus of Ota is bilaterial, mucosal and conjunctival pigmentation is usually seen. Table 21-1 compares these lesions.

Blue-brown or slate gray macules distributed symmetrically on the cheeks, forehead, temples, eyelid, or nose is characteristic of acquired bilateral nevus of Otalike macules.

Table 21-1   Bilateral Nevus of Ota Versus Bilateral Nevus of Ota-like Macules

Characteristic	Bilateral nevus of Ota	Bilateral nevus of Ota-like macules
Congenital	Often	Never
Mucosal pigmentation	Often	Never
Age of onset if acquired	All by age 30	20-70 years
Symmetric	No	Yes
Pigmentation	More intense	More subtle

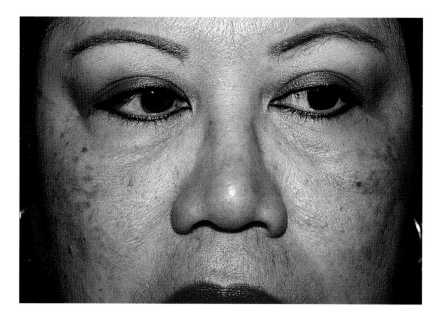

Figure 21-4   Nevus of Ota-like macules.

Histology

Melanocytes are found scattered in the upper and middermis.

Treatment

Camouflage is the usual approach to treatment of this condition. It seems likely that the same lasers effective for treatment for the nevus of Ota would be effective here, although studies documenting this have not yet been published. In one study,[7] area dermabrasion using a hand engine and a diamond fraise was performed. Of 320 patients treated, 310 (97%) achieved complete clearance of the pigment, and near complete clearance was achieved in the remaining 10 patients.

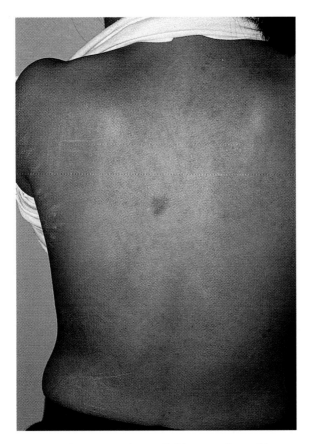

Figure 21-5   Nevus of Ito. Note the small, blue macule on this young girl's back.

NEVUS OF ITO

Clinical

A blue patch that sometimes appears to be a coalescence of macules and is unilateral on the back is characteristic of the nevus of Ito[10] (Figure 21-5). The classic lesion has its onset at birth or childhood and shows increased pigmentation in the skin innervated by the posterior supraclavicular and lateral brachial cutaneous nerves.

Treatment

It seems likely that the same lasers effective for the treatment of the nevus of Ota would be effective against the nevus of Ito, although studies documenting this have not yet been published.

MONGOLIAN SPOT

The Mongolian spot presents as a blue-black patch on the sacrum or buttocks of a neonate. Some have suggested changing the name to blue-gray macule of infancy[11] to avoid using the term *Mongolian*.

Epidemiology

The incidence of this lesion varies greatly among the races, with the darker-skinned patients being preferred. Kikuchi[12] examined 1319 3-year old Japanese children and found 95% had a residual Mongolian spot. Cordova[13] studied 437 neonates and found 96% of blacks, 46% of Hispanics, and 9.5% of whites to be affected. In another study by Alper, 89% of black, 65% of Hispanic, and only 5% of white neonates had a Mongolian spot.[14] Table 21-2 summarizes the results of these and other studies.

Etiology

Kikuchi[12] points out that 100% of newborn babies have microscopic sacral dermal melanocytes. Only in some patients are they dense enough to be clinically apparent. The question is why? What purpose do the dermal melanocytes serve? One hypothesis is that they prevent solar damage of the underlying nervous system. If this is true, one might wonder why the pigment doesn't conform more to the underlying cord and why does it fade? (Perhaps the thicker skin of older children is less easily penetrated by UV rays). Another hypothesis is that the Mongolian spot is the human version of pigmentary patterns seen in young animals such as the wild bore.[12] These spots camouflage the young animal, protecting it from being attacked or eaten.

By what process does the Mongolian spot fade? Kikuchi theorizes that as the child grows, the Mongolian spot is thinned both vertically and horizontally by the growing dermis.

Clinical

A congenital blue-black patch on the sacrum is most characteristic of a Mongolian spot (Figure 21-6). The color may be greenish-blue, blue-gray, or brown. The shape is often irregular, and the borders are indistinct. The size may range from a few millimeters to covering most of the back. Although the sacrum and buttocks are affected most often, the upper back, shoulders, or extremities are also potential sites (Figure 21-7). The color often reaches a peak at 1 to 2 years of age and then begins to fade. The majority of these lesions are gone by adolescence, although in one study of 9996 Japanese men, 4.1% had a persistent lesion and the buttocks was the most common site.[14]

Differential Diagnosis

The diagnosis of Mongolian spot is usually obvious and a biopsy is not needed. Table 21-3 provides differential diagnoses of a blue patch. Of note, the typical blue nevus has some induration to palpation, whereas the other lesions are purely macular. However, to confuse the issue, some have used the term *macular blue nevus* to describe

Table 21-2   Incidence of the Mongolian Spot in Neonates by Race

Race	Incidence
Asian	90%-100%
Black	70%-95%
Hispanic	40%-70%
White	2%-5%

congenital, persistent blue patches outside the sacral area. Rarely, a Mongolian spot is misdiagnosed as representing the sequelae of trauma (e.g., child abuse).

Histology

Histologic examination of a Mongolian spot shows elongated, dendritic, melanin-containing cells scattered lightly throughout the dermis.

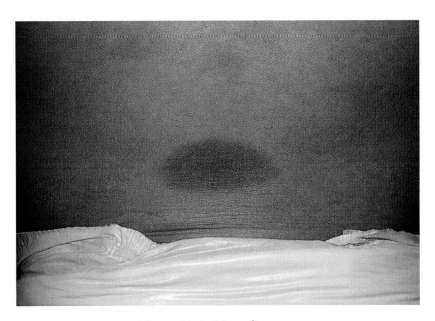

Figure 21-6   Mongolian spot.

Table 21-3   Differential Diagnosis of Blue Patches

Lesion	Onset	Typical location	Tendency to fade
Mongolian spot	Congenital	Sacrococcygeal	Yes
Nevus of Ito	Congenital or acquired	Shoulders and neck	No
Nevus of Ota	Congenital or acquired	V1 and/or V2 areas of the trigeminal nerve of the face	No
Acquired bilateral nevus of Ota-like macules	Fourth or fifth decade	Bilaterally on the forehead, temples, and malar areas	No
Dermal melanocytic hamartoma (also called *macular blue nevus* or *aberrant Mongolian spot*)	Congential	Anywhere besides the sacrum	No
Cleft lip Mongolian spot	Congenital	Upper lip	No
Late-onset dermal melanosis: an upper back variant	Fourth to sixth decade	Upper back	No

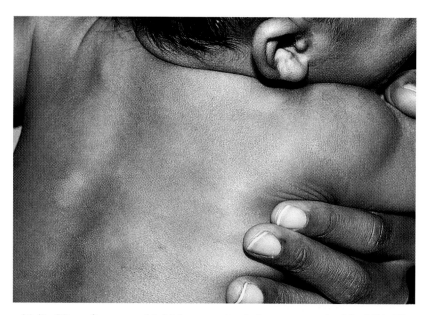

Figure 21-7   Mongolian spots. Multiple, extensive lesions are seen in this child. They were congenital and fixed.

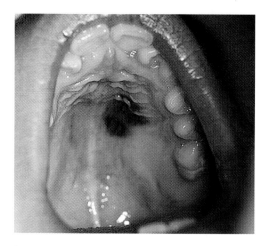

Figure 21-8   Mucosal pigmentation. This congenital blue patch was not associated with any other abnormality.

Treatment

No treatment is needed for this benign condition.

DERMAL MELANOCYTIC HAMARTOMA

Some have applied the term *aberrant Mongolian spots* to dermal melanocytic lesions occurring outside the lumbosacral area. Other terms are *dermal melanocytic hamartoma, congenital segmental dermal melanocytosis,*[15] and *macular blue nevus.* Of course, in the appropriate locations, the nevi of Ota or Ito must be considered. Isolated dermal pigmentation may occur in the oral mucosa as well (Figure 21-8). It seems to be true that blue spots localized to the sacral region tend to fade, whereas those found elsewhere tend to persist.

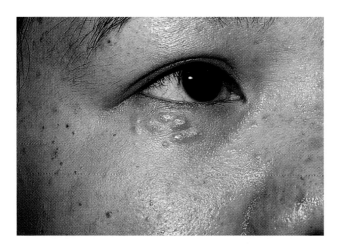

Figure 21-9   Syringomas.

Finally, the term *phakomatosis pigmentovascularis* describes the rare situation of an infant affected by both dermal melanocytic lesions and port-wine stains with or without CALSs or nevus spilus.[16]

CLEFT LIP MONGOLIAN SPOT

Clinical

A cleft lip may rarely be associated with a blue macule of the lip in a Japanese child. Mori et al[17] reported five children so affected in 1975. These pigmented lesions were in the skin and not the mucosa, were 3 to 4 mm in size, macular, bright blue to faint gray, and either sharply or diffusely marginated. Igawa et al[18] reported a much larger series from Japan. Out of 66 babies with unilateral cleft lip, 36 (55%) had a cleft lip Mongolian spot. No infant with a microform cleft lip (actual cleft does not extend beyond the vermillion border) was affected. Thus if the cleft extends beyond the vermillion border in a Japanese infant, the incidence of a blue spot is high. Of note, blue nevi may occur on the upper lip unassociated with a cleft lip.[19]

A cleft lip may rarely be associated with a blue macule of the lip in a Japanese child.

LATE-ONSET DERMAL MELANOSIS: AN UPPER BACK VARIANT

Seven elderly Japanese men have been described with the onset in middle to old age of blue macules on their upper backs.[20] The individual macules were 4 to 7 mm in size, distributed mainly in the interscapular region, and at times took on a reticulate pattern. Histology showed spindle-shaped or oval, pigment-laden cells in the dermis. No treatment is needed.

SYRINGOMAS

Clinical

Multiple flesh-colored papules on the lower eyelids and upper cheek are characteristic of syringomas (Figure 21-9). Multiple family members may be affected.

Treatment

The scarring from treatment may be worse than the appearance of the lesions. Electrosurgery and the CO_2 laser have been used.

PRURIGO PIGMENTOSA

Clinical

The sudden onset of intensely pruritic, erythematous papules that within weeks leave a reticulated pattern of hyperpigmentation is characteristic of prurigo pigmentosa. (Figure 21-10). Prurigo pigmentosa usually affects the trunk, neck, and antecubital fossae, and is most common in the Japanese, especially young women in the spring and summer. It appears that many of the cases are caused by ketosis, typically related to fasting, dieting, loss of appetite from stress, or insulin-dependant diabetes mellitus. Recent weight loss is typical. Serum or urinary ketones are typically elevated. Histologic examination shows a lichenoid inflammatory infiltrate with epidermal edema and pigmentary incontinence.

Treatment

Stopping the dieting, initiating insulin therapy, or otherwise correcting the ketosis clears the skin. In the past, before the cause of the disease was known, minocycline[3] was tried.

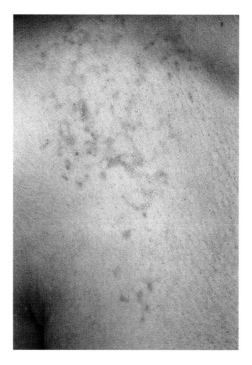

Figure 21-10   Prurigo pigmentosa.

REFERENCES

1. Nik NA, Glew WB, Zimmerman LE: Malignant melanoma of the choroid in the nevus of Ota in a black patient, *Arch Ophthalmol* 100:1641-1643, 1982.
2. Balmaceda CM et al: Nevus of Ota and leptomeningeal melanocytic lesions, *Neurology* 43:381-386, 1993.
3. Goldberg DJ, Nychay SG: Q-switched ruby laser treatment of nevus of Ota, *J Dermatol Surg Oncol* 18:817-821, 1992.
4. Lowe NJ et al: Nevus of Ota: treatment with high energy fluences of the Q-switched ruby laser, *J Am Acad Dermatol* 29:997-1001, 1993.
5. Watanabe S, Takahashi H: Treatment of nevus of Ota with the Q-switched ruby laser, *N Engl J Med* 331:1745-1750, 1994.
6. Hata Y et al: Treatment of nevus Ota: combined skin abrasion and carbon dioxide snow method, *Plast Reconstr Surg* 97:544, 1996.
7. Kunachak S et al: Dermabrasion is an effective treatment for acquired bilateral nevus of Ota-like macules, *J Dermatol Surg Oncol* 22:559-562, 1996.
8. Hori Y, Kawashimi M. Kukita A: Acquired, bilateral nevus of Ota-like macules, *J Am Acad Dermatol* 10:961-964, 1984.
9. Hidano A and reply by Hori Y: Acquired, bilateral nevus of Ota-like macules, *J Am Acad Dermatol* 12:368-369, 1985.
10. Hidano A, Kajima H, Endo Y: Bilateral nevus Ota associated with nevus Ito, *Arch Dermatol* 91:357-365, 1965.
11. Lin AE, Feingold M: Out, out damn spot, or the demise of the Mongolian spot, *Am J Dis Child* 147:714, 1993.
12. Kikuchi I: The biological significance of the Mongolian spot, *Int J Dermatol* 28:513-514, 1989.
13. Cordova A: The Mongolian spot, *Clin Pediatr* 20:714-719, 1981.
14. Hidano A: Persistent Mongolian spot in the adult, *Arch Dermatol* 103:680-681, 1971.
15. Velez A et al: Congenital segmental dermal melanocytosis in an adult, *Arch Dermatol* 128:521-525, 1992.
16. Hasegawa Y, Yasuhara M: Phakomatosis pigmentovascularis type Iva, *Arch Dermatol* 121:651-655, 1985.
17. Mori T et al: Cleft lip nevus, Jpn J Plast Reconstr Surg 18:526-527, 1975; as reported in Inoue S, Kikuchi I, Ono T: Dermal melanocytosis associated with cleft lip, *Arch Dermatol* 118:443-444, 1982.
18. Igawa HH et al: Cleft lip mongolian spot: Mongolian spot associated with cleft lip, *J Am Acad Dermatol* 30:566-569, 1994.
19. Kikuchi I, Inoue S: Common blue nevus of the upper lip—a possible relationship to Mongolian spot, *J Dermatol* 13:301-303, 1986.
20. Ono T et al: Late onset dermal melanocytosis: an upper back variant, *J Dermatol* 18:97-103, 1991.

TREATMENT

Chapter 22

Cosmetic Surgery

Daniel P. Taheri, Vic Narurkar, and Ronald L. Moy
Rhinoplasty Section: *Larry Seifert*

lthough 75% to 80% of this planet's people are nonwhites, the majority of the
cosmetic surgical literature is limited to the treatment of whites. The fear of increased pigmentary and scarring complications has made cosmetic surgeons in
the United States hesitant to perform elective procedures on both blacks and Asians.
This fear should be replaced by knowledge of unique racial differences and modifications of surgical technique to accommodate nonwhites who desire cosmetic surgery.

Understanding and accepting the attitudes of different cultures are extremely important for the cosmetic surgeon. Cultural traditions and resistance often have a pro-
found psychologic influence on the nonwhite person who is contemplating cosmetic
surgery. Changing ethnic appearance (e.g., "Westernization" of the Asian eyelid or reduction cheiloplasty in blacks) can cause feelings of guilt. Because elders play a dominant role in many nonwhite societies, their acceptance or rejection of cosmetic procedures has a psychologic influence on the ethnic patient. Altering shape while preserving
the ethnicity of the nonwhite patient is a challenge to the cosmetic surgeon.

DIFFERENCES BETWEEN PIGMENTED AND WHITE SKIN TYPES

The surgeon who contemplates performing procedures in nonwhite patients
should have an understanding of the morphologic differences between white and non-
white skin, specifically in patients of black and Asian descent. The most apparent difference between white skin and black skin is the amount of epidermal melanin.[1] Although there is no difference in the quantity of melanocytes between the two groups,
the concentration of melanin within the melanosomes is increased in black skin compared with white skin. In addition, the degradation rate of melanosomes within the
keratinocytes of black skin is slower than that of white skin. Although the increased
melanin affords protection from the harmful effects of ultraviolet light, both the
melanocytes and mesenchyma in black skin seem to be more vulnerable to trauma and
inflammatory conditions than those in white skin. Posttraumatic or postinflammatory
dyspigmentation can take the form of either hyperpigmentation or hypopigmentation.
Increased mesenchymal reactivity can result in hypertrophic scars or keloids.[1]

The stratum corneum in black skin has a similar thickness to the same layer in
white skin, but the number of layers of cells and lipid content differ. The stratum
corneum in black skin has a greater number of cell layers, as well as a higher lipid content than that of white skin. In addition, the reactivity of blood vessels is decreased in
black skin, leading to less apparent erythematous reactions after chemical exposure.[2]
These differences are important when considering chemical peels and laser resurfacing
in black patients.

Although Asian skin is classically described as having a yellowish hue, a spectrum of colors and textures exist in this population. In general, Asians that live closer to the equator will have darker skin than those who live in Northern Asia. The classic yellowish hue of Northern Chinese, Koreans, and Japanese is the result of both the number and distribution of the melanosomes rather than a difference in lipoproteins in the skin. All variations of Asian skin have a higher rate of melanin production and pigmented dermatoses. They also have a lower rate of skin malignancies than whites.[3]

Asian and black skin have a thicker dermis than white skin. Similar to black skin, Asian skin (even the lighter variations) has a greater tendency toward hypertrophic scarring.

Asian and black skin have a thicker dermis than white skin, the thickness being proportional to the intensity of pigmentation. This increased dermal thickness may account for a lower incidence in facial rhytids in Asians and blacks. Similar to black skin, Asian skin (even the lighter variations) has a greater tendency toward hypertrophic scarring. Asians may also have a greater tendency toward prolonged redness during scar maturation than white skin.[3]

Although the biochemical content of hair is similar among races, structural variations do exist.[4] In general, blacks have flat, elliptical hair follicles. Their hair is spiral-shaped and has the comparatively smallest cross sectional area. Asians have round hair follicles with straight hair. Their hair has the largest mean cross sectional area. The characteristics of the hair in whites is between that of Asians and blacks. Whites have ovoid hair follicles, wavy hair, and an intermediate-sized cross sectional area. The elliptical shape of the hair follicles in blacks predisposes them to ingrown hairs and necessitates modifications in hair transplant techniques.

RHINOPLASTY
Larry Seifert

It it generally conceded that rhinoplasty is the most difficult of aesthetic operative procedures and that rhinoplasty for the ethnic nose is particularly difficult. The surgeon is challenged by anatomic features, including the following:
1. A wide, bulbous tip with poor tip-defining points
2. Thick skin
3. Flimsy and weak tip cartilages that limit tip projection
4. Low dorsum and radix
5. Wide alar base
6. A drooping tip in the Latino nose
7. Columella retrusion
8. Foreshortened nasal length, especially in the Asian nose
9. Limited amount of available nasal septum for grafts

Added to these challenges may be psychologic considerations unique to the consideration of a change in anthropometrics that may be perceived as rejection of cultural ethnicity. The patient may ask, "Is it all right to want features similar to the Caucasian nose or will it be seen as rejecting one's heritage?" This is a very sensitive issue with strong psychologic undercurrents. The surgeon frequently hears, "I want my nose refined, but I don't want to lose who I am." The balance between desired goals and unwanted "radical" changes must be clearly defined preoperatively. Preoperative sketches, drawings, and photographs with patient anthropometric measurements are of great benefit. Usually, the patient desires a more sculpted and defined tip, with projection and tip angles. The plunging tip in the Hispanic nose requires elevation, while the short, lobular base of columella distance in the black and Asian nose demands a tip stand-up.

Open rhinoplasty is the technique of choice for the ethnic nose (Figs. 22-1 to 22-4). It offers an unparalleled view of the tip cartilages and their complex anatomic interrelationships and facilitates precise surgical adjustments. Advantages offered by open rhinoplasty include the following:
1. Suture immobilization of intercrural columellar struts
2. Precise tip grafts placement with stitch fixation
3. Reduction of widened domal cartilage segments
4. Manipulation of middle crura with interdomal sutures.

Open rhinoplasty is the technique of choice for the ethnic nose.

Septal cartilage is the graft of choice (Box 22-1). It is composed of stiff, hyaline cartilage, which yields stronger grafts for tip support and definition. Fibroelastic ear

Text continued on p. 256

Box 22-1 Flow Sheet for Tip and Dorsal Grafts

1. Septal columellar struts
   Septum: 24 mm × 4 mm
   Ear: spiral graft of concha cavum, cymba, and one third transverse bar, 24 mm × 4 mm
   Partial thickness rib cartilage: 6th and 7th ribs, harvested with gouge
2. Tip grafts
   Septum: frequently, multiple tip grafts are needed, about 10 mm × 7 mm
   Auricular
3. Dorsum
   Septum: 28 to 30 mm, alone or with sutured auricular grafts as a "sandwich" for bulk
   Auricular: bilateral conchal cartilages of 15 mm each, sutured tongue in groove
   Rib: parital thickness harvested with gouge, 30 mm × 5 mm, from flat portion 6th and 7th ribs (risk of curvature and warp)
   Bone: calvarial (hard to sculpt, risk of reabsorption)
   Soft tissue fillers for minor defects: dermis, deep temporal fascia SMASS, freeze dried human dermis; can also use these to line dorsal grafts and minimize irregularities
   Alloplasts: not for secondary nasal reconstruction; useful in Asian nose for dorsal augmentation, sutured to cartilage tip grafts and strut
Alar base modification is frequently beneficial. However, tip elevation by 4 to 5 mm with strut and dorsal cap grafts will give some reduction to the alar base width. Alar rim retraction in the region of the middle crus that occurs after tip elevation can require alar composite grafts.

SMASs, Submuscular aponeurotic systems.

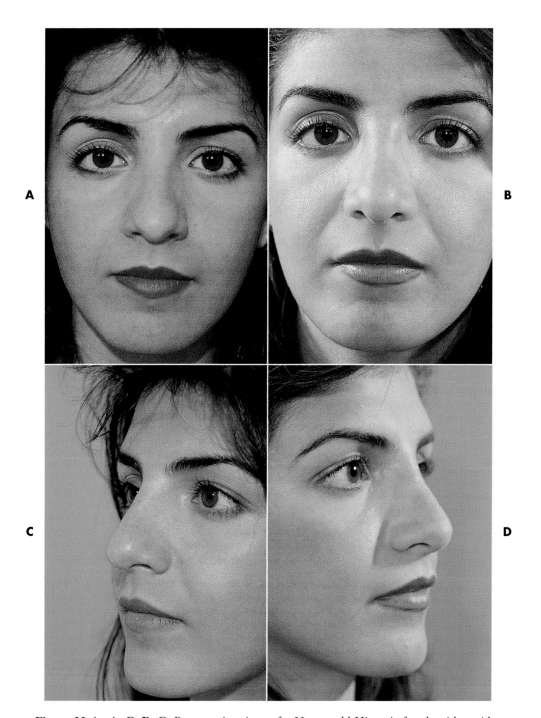

Figure 22-1   A, C, E, G, Preoperative views of a 23 year-old Hispanic female with a wide, bulbous nasal tip. **B, D, F, H,** 11-month postoperative views after open rhinoplasty with septal strut, tip graft, partial resection of domal part of middle crus, and interdomal sutures. **D,** Note elevation of tip, improved alar-columellar relationship, and correction of columellar retrusion with strut. **G,** Preoperative worm's-eye view. Note the lack of tip projection and definition. **H,** Note inconspicuous columellar scar.

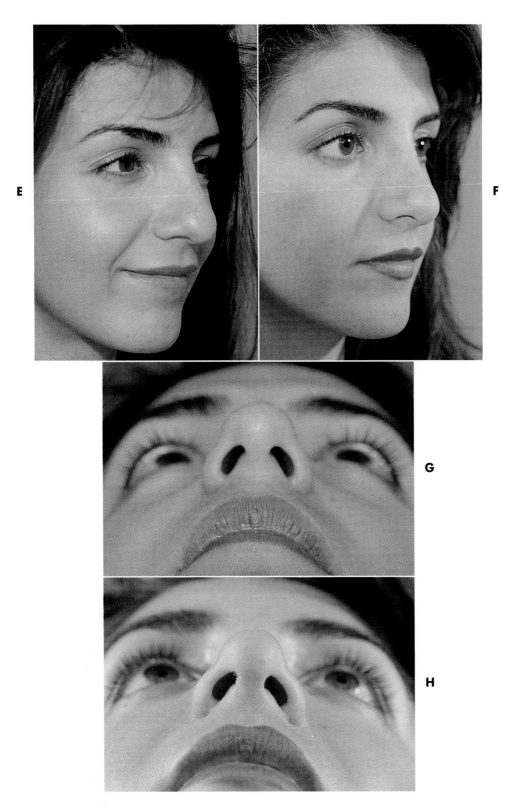

Figure 22-1, cont'd   For legend see opposite page.

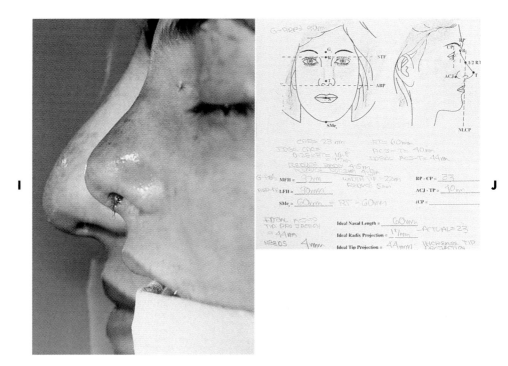

Figure 22-1, cont'd   I, Intraoperative view. Note improved tip aesthetics compared with the preoperative view and the tip breakpoint angles achieved by strut and tip graft. **J,** Preoperative worksheet with anthropometric analysis. A 4 mm tip elevation was calculated and achieved by tip graft, strut, and middle crus suture modification.

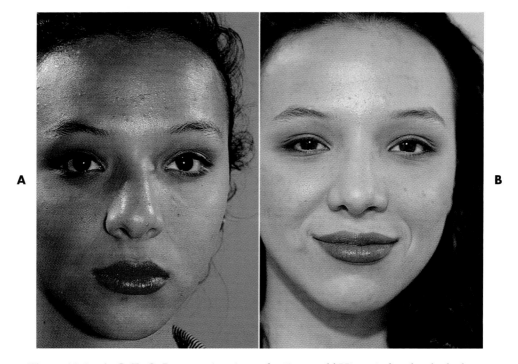

Figure 22-2   A, C, E, G, Preoperative views of a 19 year-old Hispanic female who had open rhinoplasty with tip reduction and suture modification, septal columellar strut 24 mm × 4 mm, and tip graft. **B, D, F, H,** 1-year postoperative views.

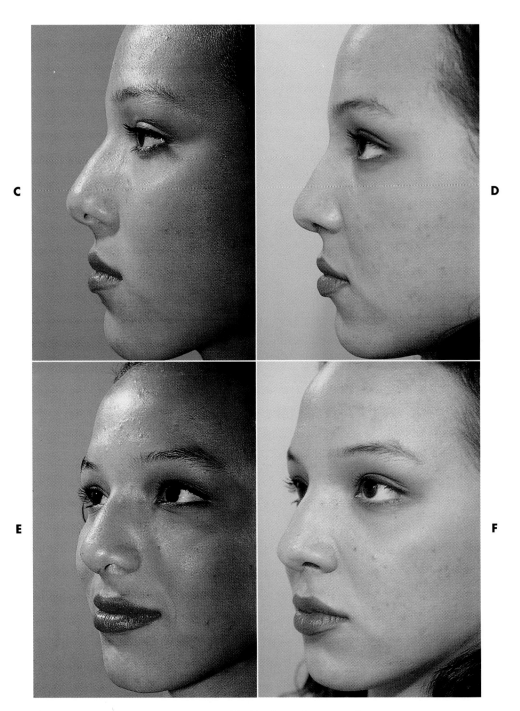

Figure 22-2, cont'd   For legend see opposite page.   *Continued*

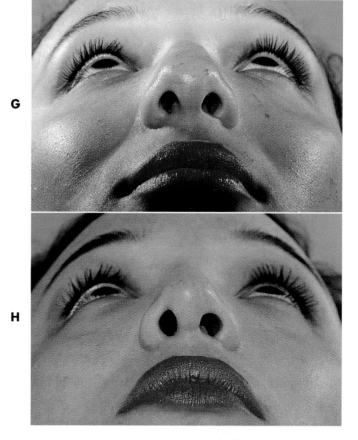

Figure 22-2, cont'd   For legend see p. 250.

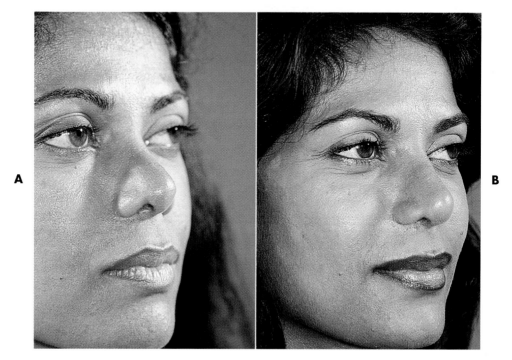

Figure 22-3   **A, C, G,** Preoperative views of a 37-year-old Indian female with two previous closed, endonasal rhinoplasties. Note the foreshortened nose, the alar base scarring, concave dorsum, low nasal radix, and the lack of tip projection. Reconstruction was done with septal cartilage bilateral auricular cartilage grafts and compound auricular graft. **B,** 1-year postoperative view after open rhinoplasty with dorsal reconstruction with septal and auricular cartilage graft. The nose is lengthened with dorsal nasal and tip grafts. The alar rim cephalic retraction is improved by auricular composite graft (see **E**).

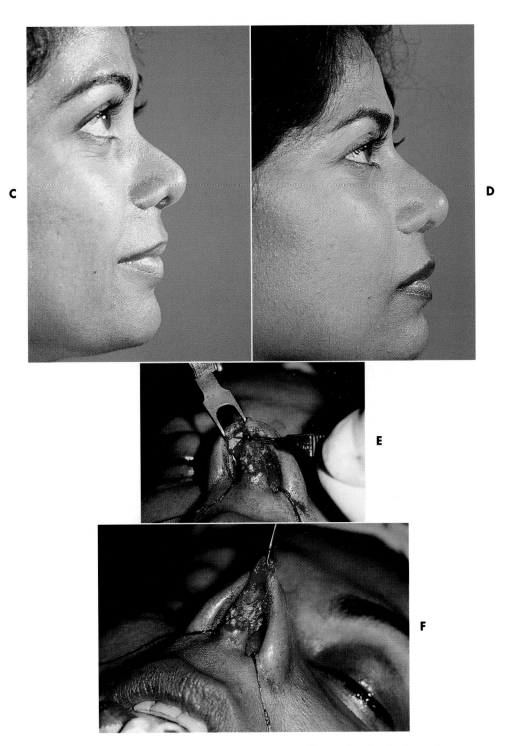

Figure 22-3, cont'd D, Dorsal and tip augmentation with septal and auricular grafts at postoperative follow-up. **E,** Note the tip graft sutured to the strut. The forceps point to the auricular composite graft to improve alar rim retraction. **F,** Intraoperative view. Note tip graft sutured to strut. The columellar skin is advanced 3 mm by undermining to anterior nasal spine and rotated as an advancement flap to gain soft tissue length.

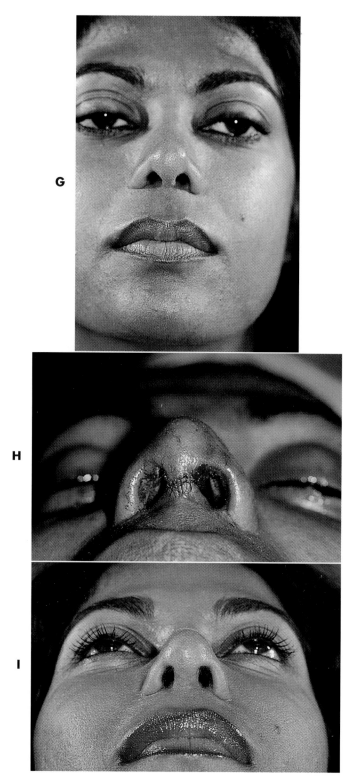

Figure 22-3, cont'd   G, Note the alar base scars and wide, full, rounded tip without tip-defining points. **H,** Intraoperative view. Note the tip projection of 4 to 5 mm. The alar bases are narrowed 3 mm as the tip and lobule are elevated by strut and graft. **I,** Note the inconspicuous scar, the tip elevation, and the narrowing of alar bases by elevation of the tip and lobule without further alar base modification.

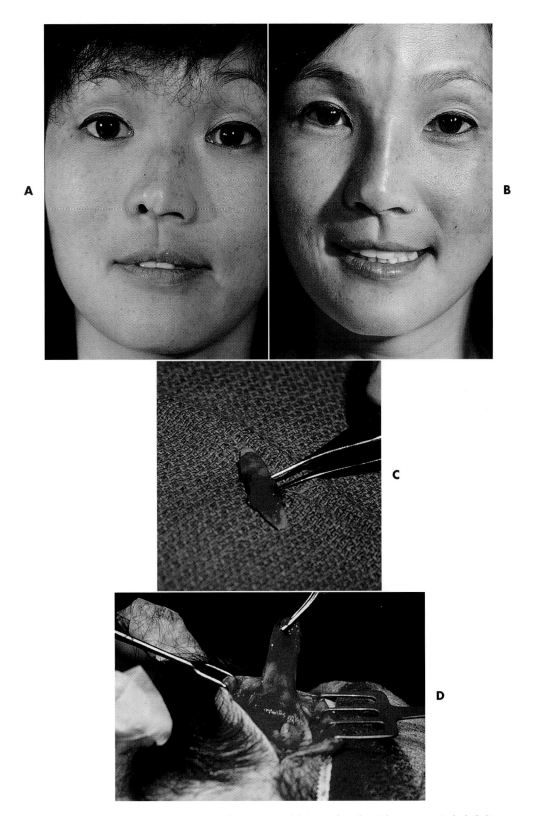

Figure 22-4 **A,** Preoperative view of a 32-year-old Asian female with a congenital cleft-lip-like nasal deformity with shallow nasal dorsum and unsupported asymmetric alar rims and lower lateral cartilages. **B,** 4-month postoperative view. A closed endonasal rhinoplasty was done using a partial thickness autogenous rib cartilage graft harvested by a gouge from the 7th rib. The rib cartilage graft was covered with temporalis fascia. **C,** Rib cartilage graft covered with temporalis fascia; note minimal curvature. **D,** Deep temporalis fascia harvested to cover the rib cartilage to minimize irregularities.

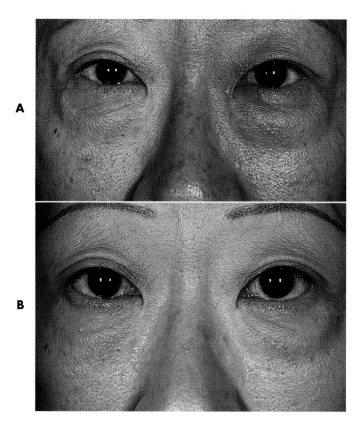

Figure 22-5   Preoperative **(A)** and postoperative **(B)** blepharoplasty views of an Asian patient.

cartilage is flimsy compared with hyaline septal cartilage and is less well suited for tip-defining grafts.

BLEPHAROPLASTY

Knowledge of the anatomic differences between the upper eyelids of whites and Asians is necessary for performing blepharoplasty in Asians. Absence of the superior palpebral fold produces a "single eyelid" appearance in approximately 50% of the Asian population. Asians without a superior palpebral fold lack the dermal attachments between the levator aponeurosis and/or the tarsal plate that are responsible for the crease in the upper eyelids of whites. The periorbital fat in Asians is more abundant than in the eyelids of whites, extending inferiorly anterior to the tarsal plate. The lack of the superior palpebral fold, excess skin, and abundance of periorbital fat contribute to the characteristic puffiness of the Asian upper eyelid (Figure 22-5). The epicanthal fold is a web of skin over the medial canthus and is present in approximately 90% of the upper eyelids of Asians. The size and shape of the epicanthal fold are highly variable, and therefore several different techniques are available for modification of the epicanthal fold.[5]

When discussing blepharoplasty with Asian patients, the size and shape of the new eyelid and the modification of the epicanthal fold should be ascertained. Many patients are very particular about the shape of the eyelid (round versus oval) and whether the new superior palpebral fold should be continuous with the epicanthal fold ("inside fold") or extend medial to the epicanthal fold ("outside fold").

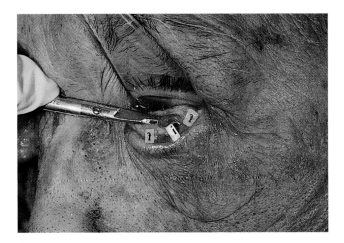

Figure 22-6 Intraoperative view of blepharoplasty.

Technical modifications of procedures commonly used on white patients include the following:

1. Creation of a superior palpebral fold by skin excision and fixation sutures to the levator aponeurosis to form a "double eyelid"
2. Excision of the central and lateral periorbital fat pads (Figure 22-6)
3. Epicanthoplasty by simple advancement, half Z-plasty, or W-plasty

Complications are not uncommon with blepharoplasty in Asians; up to 10% will require revision procedures. Complications that are of special concern with blepharoplasty in Asians include eyelid asymmetry, loss of the palpebral fold, laxity of pretarsal skin, retraction of the upper eyelid, hypertrophic scars, and excessive fat removal.[3]

Complications that are of special concern with blepharoplasty include in Asians eyelid asymmetry, loss of the palpebral fold, laxity of pretarsal skin, retraction of the upper eyelid, hypertrophic scars, and excessive fat removal.

KELOIDS

The keloid should be treated so that the involved anatomic region is functional and cosmetically acceptable. Additionally, the intervention must be such that the keloid does not recur. Surgical excision of keloids has a 55% recurrence rate.[6,7] When possible, simple excision is the best alternative. The use of tension-reducing measures such as Z-plasty is not recommended because it may extend the keloid. The excision should be performed with sharp instruments to inflict the least amount of trauma during the procedure. The number of sutures should also be limited because foreign body reactions increase the possibility of keloidal regrowth. On the earlobes, it is best to avoid the use of buried, absorbable sutures and use only nonabsorbable skin sutures that have low reactivity.

The number of sutures should also be limited because foreign body reactions increase the possibility of keloidal regrowth.

When simple excision is not an option because of excessive skin tension, the use of skin grafts or flaps may be considered. Some investigators have advocated an auto-grafting procedure in which the epidermis overlying the keloid is dissected. The bulk of the keloid is then removed, and the epidermis is then placed over the defect.[8,9] This technique is especially useful for the removal of large keloids. Although a full-thickness graft may be superior to this split-thickness graft, it is likely that the full-thickness graft would be less likely to lead to keloid formation because of the intact microvasculature in the reticular dermis.[10] The disadvantage of this technique would be the possibility of keloid formation at the donor site.

A number of adjunctive treatments have been reported in the literature to improve the results of keloid removal. These modalities include intralesional steroid injections, cryotherapy, laser surgery, pressure dressings, topical silicone sheetings, and radio-therapy.

The use of intralesional steroid injections in the treatment of keloids was origi-nally introduced by Maguire in 1965.[11] A very useful adjunctive treatment modality, the injections may be used as the sole treatment[14] or may be used in combination with other techniques.[12-14] Corticosteroids act via two mechanisms: they decrease the syn-thesis of collagen while increasing the degradation of collagen.[15-17] Presurgical, in-tralesional injection of corticosteroids at least 1 month before the excision in combi-nation with repeated postsurgical administration of corticosteroids has been advocated. This includes monthly triamcinolone (Kenalog) injections for 6 months after the surgery, with less frequent injections thereafter.[18] If this postoperative injection regimen is not maintained, keloids tend to recur. Additionally, the lower concentrations of steroids are ineffective in preventing keloid regrowth. Interestingly, it has been shown that a single intraoperative injection of steroids is successful in preventing the recur-rence of keloids.[19] Hypopigmentation is a common sequelae in the darker-skinned pop-ulation[20] and patients should be observed for signs of it. If discoloration does occur, it tends to fade with time.[8]

Another adjunctive modality is the use of pressure. Pressure has been shown to stop further keloid growth in the partially occluded microvasculature of hypertrophic scars.[21]

Radiotherapy is another modality that was used fairly extensively in the past[22,23] but has been mostly abandoned because of reports of complications, including thyroid cancer, many years after treatment.[24]

Another adjunctive modality in the treatment of keloids is cryotherapy. Because of melanocyte sensitivity to cold injury, there is a high risk of depigmentation when using this modality. Success rates have been variable, though impressive results have been reported by some investigators. The risk of hypopigmentation decreases signifi-cantly if cryotherapy and intralesional steroids are used conjunctively in adjuvant treat-ment of keloids.[25]

An improvement in color, texture, and induration of keloids has been reported with use of a topical silicone sheeting several hours per day.[26-28]

Laser surgery using the carbon dioxide laser was originally thought to hold great promise in the treatment of keloids. The laser seals blood vessels as it cuts and causes minimal necrosis in the surrounding tissue.[29] Subsequent studies, however, have failed to show significant advantage of the carbon dioxide laser over conventional surgery.[30,31] Preliminary studies by other investigators have reported promising results with the use of the Nd:YAG laser.[32-34]

To achieve the best resolution of the keloid, the use of combined modalities with an observation period of at least 2 years is necessary to effectively limit the possibility of recurrence. Although treatment of keloids presents a difficult problem, a significant improvement in cosmesis may be achieved.

HAIR TRANSPLANTS

Male-pattern hair loss in blacks tends to occur later in life and with a lower frequency compared with whites. Although less common on the scalp, the potential for development of postsurgical keloids warrants a higher level of caution before proceeding with hair transplants. Performance of a test graft followed by a waiting period of 3 months before proceeding with the entire procedure has been advocated.[35] Because of the texture and curve of the hair shaft in blacks, fewer grafts are needed to create the illusion of greater hair density.[36] Adding saline to the donor site will help to straighten the follicles and thus provide more viable hairs for transplantation.[35,37] Another minor modification in technique is to use larger (4 mm) punch grafts and manually remove the grafts to prevent transection of hair follicles and to produce more viable hairs. In white patients, satisfactory results are obtained with smaller punches and mechanical removal of grafts.[38]

The potential for development of postsurgical keloids warrants a higher level of caution before proceeding.

CHEILOPLASTY

Often, the patient desiring rhinoplasty will overlook the retruded chin, and the surgeon will neglect the value of lip reduction to improve the result of rhinoplasty and menoplasty. Pierce[38] has advocated the importance of analyzing the nose, chin, and lip complex in the black patient. Reduction cheiloplasty is a simple technique that involves removing a 1 to 2 cm strip of mucosa with minor salivary glands posterior to the wet line of the lip. Stucker[39] reviewed the photographs of 100 black patients who had undergone rhinoplasty and found that 50% would have benefited from a reduction cheiloplasty.

SCLEROTHERAPY

The incidence of superficial ectatic venules in blacks and whites is the same. No differences in postsclerotherapy complications and side effects have been reported between blacks and whites.[40] No significant increase in the frequency of postsclerotherapy hyperpigmentation in pigmented skin as compared with white skin has been reported. A similar outcome as a result of treatment would be expected regardless of skin phototype.

CHEMICAL PEELS

Although chemical peel is an established technique for improving wrinkles and acne scarring and correcting pigmentary disorders such as melasma and postinflammatory hyperpigmentation, caution should be exercised in performing a chemical peel on a pigmented patient. There is limited data confirming the safety and efficacy of this procedure on postinflammatory changes and melasma in black patients.[41-43] Cutaneous melanocytes respond unpredictably to trauma, and numerous instances of pigmentary change have been reported after chemical peels. In general, in darker skin phototypes, phenol peels may induce areas of depigmentation and hypopigmentation. Additionally, deeper peels may also cause keloid formation. In contrast, the more superficial peels (such as Jessner's and glycolic acid peels) tend to cause hyperpigmentation.[44] This pigmentary change exaggerates the difference between treated and untreated skin, thereby emphasizing the need for feathering of the edges. The other side effects, including posttreatment infection, milia, and enlarged pores, occur with the same frequency regardless of the skin phototype.

DERMABRASION

Although being replaced by laser resurfacing, dermabrasion is still commonly used in the treatment of wrinkles and acne scarring. Many investigators have reported disappointing results with dermabrasion used in the treatment of pigmented skin. Initial hypopigmentation over the first month, followed by hyperpigmentation, is a common complication of the procedure.[44] This hyperpigmentation may be more noticeable in lighter-skinned blacks.[44] Patients should be advised to reduce exposure to sunlight for 6 months after dermabrasion because such exposure will contribute to alterations in pigmentation. Corrective cosmetics may be used to camouflage the depigmented areas.

LIPOSUCTION

Body contouring surgery via suction-assisted removal of fat is a well-established technique. Although similar techniques are used regardless of the ethnic origin of the patient, dysmorphic obesity has a special preference for certain people. The different tendencies to develop adipose deposits have been described as follows[1]: Hispanics have a tendency to develop rolls on the hips with a short and inverted subgluteal crease. Whites develop hip rolls in continuity with an abdominal roll. Fat deposits in Asians extend from the waist to the chest and arms. Undesirable complications do not differ, except for a slightly higher rate of keloids and hypertrophic scars at the site of cannula insertion and hyperpigmentation over the treated sites in blacks.

REFERENCES

1. Grimes PE, Hunt SG: Considerations for cosmetic surgery in the black population, *Clin Plast Surg* 20(1):27, 1993.
2. Berardesca E, Maibach HI: Sensitive and ethnic skin: a need for special skin care agents, *Dermatol Clin* 9:89, 1991.
3. McCurdy JA: Cosmetic surgery of the Asian face, New York, 1990, Theime Medical Publishers.
4. Grimes PE, Davis LT: Cosmetics in blacks, *Dermatol Clin* 9:53, 1991.
5. McCurdy JA: Blepharoplasty in the oriental eye, *Am J Cosmetic Surg* 2:29, 1985.
6. Borges AF, Alexander JE: Relaxed skin tension lines, Z-plasties on scars and fusiform excision of lesions, *Br J Plast Surg* 15:242, 1962.
7. Cosman B, Wolff M: Correlation of keloid recurrence with completeness of local excision, *Plast Reconst Surg* 50:163-165, 1972.
8. Pollack SV, Goslen JB: The surgical treatment of keloids, *J Dermatol Surg Oncol* 8:1045-1049, 1982.
9. Apfelberg DB, Maser MR, Lash H: The use of epidermis over a keloid as an autograft after resection of the keloid, *J Dermatol Surg Oncol* 2:409-11, 1976.
10. Salasche SJ, Grabski WJ: Keloids of the earlobes: a surgical technique, *J Dermatol Surg Oncol* 9:552-556, 1983.

11. Maguire HC: Treatment of keloids with triamcinolone acetonide injected intralesionally, *JAMA* 192:325-327, 1965.
12. Pierce HE: Keloids: enigma of the plastic surgeon, *J Natl Med Assn* 71:1177-1180, 1979.
13. Ketchum LD, Cohen IK, Masters FW: Hypertrophic scars and keloids, *Plast Reconstr Surg* 53:140-154, 1974.
14. Hirshowitz B, Lerner D, Moscona AR: Treatment of keloid scars by combined cryosurgery and intralesional corticosteroids, *Anesthetic Plast Surg* 61:153-158, 1982.
15. Diegelmann RE, Bryant CP, Cohen IK: Tissue alpha globulins in keloid formation, *Plast Reconst Surg* 59:418, 1977.
16. Cohen IK, Diegelmann RF: The biology of keloids and hypertrophic scars and the influence of corticosteroids, *Clin Plast Surg* 4:297-299, 1977.
17. McCoy BJ, Diegelmann RF, Cohen IK: Effect of triamcinolone acetonide on collagen synthesis and prolyl-hydroxylase activity by keloid and normal skin fibroblasts, *Fed Proc* 38:818, 1979.
18. Brown LA, Pierce HE: Keloids: scar revision, *J Dermatol Surg Oncol* 12(1):51-56, 1986.
19. Golladay ES: Treatment of keloids by single intraoperative perilesional injection of repository steroid, *South Med J* 81:736-738, 1988.
20. Oluwasanmi JO: Keloids in the African, *Clin Plast Surg* 1:179-195, 1974.
21. Kischer CW, Shetlar MR: Microvasculature in hypertrophic scars and the effects of pressure, *J Trauma*, 19:757-764, 1979.
22. Ollstein RN et al: Treatment of keloids by combined excision and immediate postoperative x-ray therapy, *Ann Plast Surg* 7:281-285, 1981.
23. Levy DS, Salter MM, Roth RE: Postoperative irradiation in the prevention of keloids, *Am J Roentgenol* 127:509-510, 1976.
24. Hoffman S: Radiotherapy for keloids? *Ann Plast Surg* 9:265, 1982.
25. Quinn KJ: Silicone gel in scar treatment, *Burns* 13:S33-S40, 1987.
26. Mercer NS: Silicone gel in the treatment of keloid scars, *Br J Plast Surg* 42:83-87, 1989.
27. Murdoch ME, Salisbury JA, Gibson JR: Silicone gel in the treatment of keloids, *Acta Derm Venereol* 70:181-183, 1990.
28. Hirshowitz B, Lerner D, Moscona AR: Treatment of keloid scars by combined cryosurgery and intralesional corticosteroids, *Anesthetic Plast Surg* 61:153-158, 1982.
29. Wheeland RG, Bailin PL: Dermatologic application of the argon and carbon dioxide lasers, *Current Concepts in Skin Disorders*, Summer 1984, p 5.
30. Stern JC, Lucente FE: Carbon dioxide laser excision of earlobe keloids: a prospective study and critical analysis of existing data, *Arch Otolaryngol Head Neck Surg* 115:1107-1111, 1989.
31. Apfelberg DB et al: Failure of carbon dioxide laser excision of keloids, *Lasers Surg Med* 9:382-388, 1989.
32. Apfelberg DB et al: Preliminary report on use of the Nd:YAG laser in plastic surgery, *Lasers Surg Med* 7:189-198, 1987.
33. Sherman R, Rosenfeld H: Experience with the Nd:YAG laser in the treatment of keloid scars, *Ann Plast Surg* 21:231-235, 1988.
34. Castro DJ et al: Bioinhibition of human fibroblast cultures sensitized to Q-switch II dye and treated with the Nd:YAG laser: a new technique of photodynamic therapy with lasers, *Laryngoscope* 99:421-428, 1989.
35. Pierce HE: *Cosmetic plastic surgery in non-white patients*, New York, 1982, Grune & Stratton, pp 70-75.
36. Unger WP: Hair replacement surgery in the black male and female. In Pierce HE: *Cosmetic plastic surgery in non-white patients*, New York, 1982, Grune & Stratton, pp 51-69.
37. Pierce HE: The uniqueness of hair transplantation in black patients. *J Dermatol Surg Oncol* 3:533-535, 1977.
38. Pierce HE: The uniqueness of hair transplantation in black patients, *J Dermatol Surg Oncol* 3:533, 1977.
39. Stucker FJ: Reduction cheiloplasty: an adjunctive procedure in the black rhinoplasty patient, *Arch Otolaryngol Head Neck Surg*, 114:779, 1988.
40. Duffy DM: Personal communication.

41. Bulengo-Ransby SM: Topical tretinoin (retinoic acid) therapy for hyperpigmented lesions caused by inflammation of the skin in black patients, *N Engl J Med* 328:1438-1443, 1993.

42. Garcia A, Fulton JE Jr: The combination of glycolic acid and hydroquinone or kojic acid for the treatment of melasma and related conditions, *Dermatol Surg* 22:443-447, 1996.

43. Grimes PE: Melasma: etiologic and therapeutic considerations, *Arch Dermatol* 131:1453-1457, 1995.

44. Pierce H, Brown L: Laminar dermal reticulopathy and chemical peeling in the black patient, *J Dermatol Surg Oncol* 12:69-73, 1980.

Chapter 23

Laser Therapy

Daniel P. Taheri, Vic Narurkar, and Ronald L. Moy

L aser therapy in pigmented skin poses several challenges. The interaction of laser light with tissue depends on chromophores to absorb incident laser light. Selective photothermolysis occurs when selective tissue absorption of laser light leads to selective destruction of the absorbing tissue.[1] In cutaneous laser surgery, the key chromophores are oxyhemoglobin, hemoglobin, and melanin. Advances in selective lasers have focused on designing laser delivery systems that are specific for the wavelengths for biologically active chromophores. In pigmented skin, interference with melanin poses significant challenges for laser therapy. This chapter will review approaches to laser therapy in pigmented skin.

PIGMENTED SKIN

The classification of skin types based on response to ultraviolet irradiation was developed by Fitzpatrick (Box 23-1). Laser therapy is safest in skin types I to III. Skin types IV to VI present significant challenges because of greater damage to melanin, resulting in hypopigmentation, hyperpigmentation, depigmentation, and streaky pigmentation.[2] The majority of cutaneous lasers have significant overlap with the absorp-

---

Box 23-1 Fitzpatrick Skin Phototypes

Type I: Always burns easily, shows no immediate pigment darkening, never tans.

Type II: Always burns easily, trace immediate pigment darkening, tans minimally and with difficulty.

Type III: Burns minimally, + immediate pigment darkening, tans gradually and uniformly (light brown).

Type IV: Burns minimally, ++ immediate pigment darkening, tans well (moderate brown).

Type V: Rarely burns, +++ immediate pigment darkening, tans very well (dark brown).

Type VI: Never burns, +++ immediate pigment darkening, tans profusely (black).

From Fitzpatrick TB: *Arch Dermatol* 124:869, 1988.

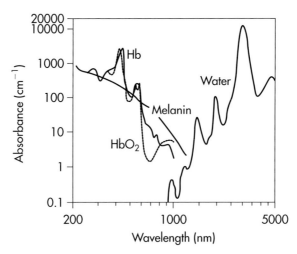

Figure 23-1 Absorption spectrum of biologically active chromophores—melanin and hemoglobin—and absorption spectrum of various laser delivery systems.

tion spectrum of melanin (Figure 23-1). Changes in pigmentation may not be apparent for several months after laser therapy. Therefore when treating pigmented skin, test sites and long-term follow-up are recommended before performing laser treatment.

OVERVIEW OF CURRENT LASER DELIVERY SYSTEMS

Current laser delivery systems can be divided based on the desired target of destruction (Table 23-1). These systems include vascular lasers, epidermal pigmented lesion lasers, dermal pigmented lesion lasers, skin resurfacing lasers, and destructive lasers for excisional surgery. Modes of laser delivery include continuous wave systems, quasi-pulsed or gated systems, and pulsed systems. Most selective laser delivery systems employ pulsed modes for delivery. Lasers in the visible light wavelength have the highest coincidental absorption with melanin and therefore carry the highest risk of changes in pigmentation, whereas lasers in the far infrared range have the lowest risk of changes in pigmentation (Table 23-1).

A variety of cutaneous conditions are more frequently encountered in pigmented skin, and some are effectively treated with laser therapy. However, many lesions that can be effectively treated with laser therapy in Fitzpatrick skin types I to III show poor response and/or greater complications in pigmented skin.

DISORDERS OF PIGMENTATION

Pigmented individuals will most often seek consultation for laser therapy to treat disorders of pigmentation. Because of epidermal and dermal components of these disorders and a higher risk of unwanted melanin injury, disorders of pigmentation are most challenging to treat.

Epidermal Pigmented Lesions (Lentigines, Ephelides, Lentigos)

Epidermal pigmented lesions can be successfully treated with the 510-nm pulsed dye laser,[3] the Q-switched Nd:YAG laser at 532 nm,[4] the copper vapor laser,[5] the Q-

Table 23-1   Overview of Available Laser Delivery Systems and Their Response in Pigmented Skin (Fitzpatrick Skin Types IV-VI)

Target	Laser	Risk of pigmentation changes
Vascular lesions	Flash-lamp pumped pulsed dye (585 nm, 590 nm, 595 nm, 600 nm)	Moderate to high
	Long pulse 532 nm	Moderate to high
	Diode 532 nm	Moderate to high
	Copper	Moderate to high
	Krypton	Moderate to high
	Argon	High
Pigmented lesions	Copper	Moderate to high
	510 nm pulsed dye	Moderate to high
	Krypton	Moderate to high
	Q-switched alexandrite	Moderate
	Q-switched Nd:YAG at 532 nm	Moderate to high
	Q-switched ruby	Moderate to high
Tattoos	Q-switched alexandrite	Moderate
	Q-switched ruby	Moderate to high
	Q-switched Nd:YAG at 1064 nm	Low
Skin resurfacing	Erbium-YAG	Moderate
	Pulsed carbon dioxide	High
Hair removal*	Long-pulse alexandrite*	Moderate
	Long-pulse ruby*	Moderate to high
	Q-switched Nd:YAG with topical suspension†	Low

*Long-term studies are underway.
†System FDA-approved for hair removal at time of publication.

switched ruby laser,[6] and the Q-switched alexandrite laser. All of these lasers carry a small risk of depigmentation and hypopigmentation in darker skin.[7] However, the laser does provide a more precise destruction with a lower chance of hyperpigmentation as compared with cryotherapy. A test area should be evaluated before treatment is initiated at a low fluence. Labial lentigines are most common in pigmented skin and have shown an excellent response to Q-switched ruby laser treatment.[8]

Melasma

Melasma may be epidermal, dermal, or mixed. The majority of melasma patients have dermal and epidermal components.[9] Wood's light examination can help determine the depth of melasma. Melasma poses one of the most challenging treatment approaches in all skin types. Laser therapy with the 510-nm pigmented lesion pulsed dye laser[10] and the Q-switched ruby laser[11] has generally been disappointing.

Laser therapy with the 510-nm pigmented lesion pulsed dye laser and the Q-switched ruby laser has generally been disappointing.

Postinflammatory Hyperpigmentation

In pigmented skin, postinflammatory hyperpigmentation is exceedingly common. As with melasma, treatment with lasers is generally disappointing. A few reports show favorable response of posttraumatic hyperpigmentation in Asian patients to treatment with the Q-switched ruby laser.[12] Postsclerotherapy hyperpigmentation has shown favorable response with the flash-lamp pumped dye laser; however, because of significant melanin overlap, the flash-lamp pumped pulse dye laser should be used with caution in darker skin.

Infraorbital Dark Circles

Infraorbital dark circles can result from melanin deposition, increased vasculature, or a combination of these factors. This condition is far more prevalent in pigmented skin. Successful treatment of melanin-induced infraorbital pigmentation has been reported with the Q-switched alexandrite laser, the Q-switched ruby laser,[13] and the Q-switched double frequency Nd:YAG laser at 1064 nm.[14] In pigmented skin, the Q-switched Nd:YAG laser poses the least risk of hypopigmentation or depigmentation. A small test area should be treated before proceeding with treatment of the entire area. Although data is lacking, resurfacing lasers may also be of benefit.

The Q-switched alexandrite and the Q-switched ruby lasers successfully clear this condition without significant scarring.

Nevus of Ota/Nevus of Ito

Dermal melanocytosis can present as nevus of Ota, a commonly found, slate-grey/bluish patch on facial skin, or nevus of Ito, which occurs on the upper extremities.[15] Nevus of Ota is commonly found in Asians and blacks and has a special preference for females, with some statistics showing the prevalence to be between 1% to 2% of the Japanese population.[16] The Q-switched alexandrite and the Q-switched ruby lasers successfully clear this condition without significant scarring.[17-19] Multiple treatments at 6- to 12-week intervals are necessary. There are no reports in the literature for the treatment of nevus of Ito, although theoretically a similar response should be expected.

Traumatic and Decorative Tattoos

Before the development of selective lasers, treatment of traumatic and decorative tattoos resulted in significant scarring. Traumatic tattoos include gunpowder tattoos, road gravel, etc. Decorative tattoos include a variety of pigments. Q-switched lasers have revolutionized treatment of tattoos. Superficial, blue-black tattoos show the best response to laser therapy with all three Q-switched lasers (alexandrite, ruby, and double-frequency Nd:YAG).[20] Green pigment is difficult to treat and shows favorable response to alexandrite and ruby lasers.[21] Red pigment shows favorable response to the Nd:YAG double-frequency laser at 532 nm.[22] Other colors have shown a favorable response to the Q-switched alexandrite laser.[22] Paradoxic darkening can occur with white ink and cosmetic tattooing such as lipliner and eyeliner, after the Q-switched laser treatment.[23]

In pigmented skin, the Q-switched double frequency Nd:YAG laser at 1064 nm is the laser of choice for treating tattoos. It has the lowest risk of causing changes in pigmentation as a result of lowest coincidental absorption with melanin.[24] Transient hypopigmentation can occur with this laser, but it is generally reversible.[24]

Vitiligo

Vitiligo poses a significant challenge for therapy in dark skin. Some anecdotal reports have shown efficacy of the Q-switched ruby laser[25-27] at wavelengths of 595 nm and 600 nm,[28] designed to treat recalcitrant vascular lesions and lower extremity spider telangiectasias. With all vascular lesions, there is significant concern for pigmentary interference with melanin, and therefore less than optimal clearance of vascular lesions in dark skin.[29] The flash-lamp pumped pulse dye laser (FPDL) carries the lowest risk of pigmentary changes as compared with other vascular lasers, but treatment of lesions such as port wine stains in dark skin (Figure 23-2) has not been reported to be very successful.[30] Pilot studies have shown promising results with the FPDL at longer pulse durations for the treatment of lower extremity spider telangiectasias.[31] However, even in Fitzpatrick skin types I to III, there is significant risk of hyperpigmentation, and the FPDL at either pulse duration does not work as well for the darker skin types. A newer variable pulse 532 nm solid state laser with a chilling tip to prevent unwanted epidermal injury is currently being investigated to overcome these limitations.[32]

Skin Resurfacing

The field of cutaneous resurfacing with lasers has witnessed unparalleled growth. The first reports of skin resurfacing were performed with carbon dioxide lasers in the superpulsed modes.[33] Because of unwanted thermal damage, results were not optimal and carried a significant risk of scarring. The development of pulsed carbon dioxide laser delivery systems and carbon dioxide lasers using optomechanical shutters to reduce tissue dwell time[34] has enabled laser skin resurfacing to gain widespread acceptance. The two most widely studied laser delivery systems are the Ultrapulse laser and Silk-Touch systems.[35] Both modes allow for selective and controlled thermal destruc-

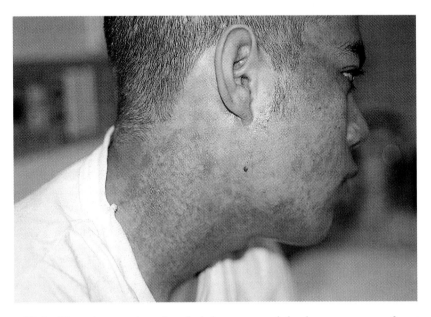

Figure 23-2 Hypopigmentation after flash-lamp pumped dye laser treatment of port–wine stain in an Asian patient.

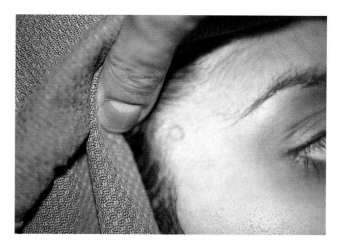

Figure 23-3   Performance of a test site and assessment at 3 to 6 months on the temporal area for skin resurfacing with the ultrapulse laser in a Hispanic patient.

tion of the epidermis and dermis without significant thermal damage to the surrounding tissue. Additional systems are currently being investigated, including carbon dioxide lasers in the microsecond domain and other wavelengths such as the Erbium-YAG laser.[36]

Indications for skin resurfacing include photoaging, rhytids, surgical scars, traumatic scars, and acne scars. Skin resurfacing is generally recommended for Fitzpatrick skin types I to III because of the risk of permanent changes in pigmentation that can ensue after thermal destruction of the epidermis and dermis.[37] In pigmented skin, the majority of requests for skin resurfacing are for acne scarring. There are a handful of reports demonstrating the efficacy of using pulsed carbon dioxide lasers for acne scarring in Asian patients.[38] Hyperpigmentation can be corrected by using bleaching agents before and after laser treatment. However, depigmentation and hypopigmentation are generally not reversible. A test site may be used when considering skin resurfacing for Fitzpatrick skin types IV and higher (Figure 23-3). This is not always a reliable predictor of posttreatment complications.

Scars, Keloids, and Striae Distensae

Lasers have been successful in the treatment of hypertrophic scars, keloids, and striae distensae. Hypertrophic scars have been successfully treated with the flash-lamp pumped pulse dye laser to improve color and texture of the scar.[39] With the FPDL, there is a risk of pigmentary change; however, the improvement in texture usually overcomes the limitations posed by any changes in pigmentation (Figure 23-4).

Hypertrophic scars have been successfully treated with the flash-lamp pumped pulse dye laser.

Keloids are distinguished from hypertrophic scars by their tendency to spread beyond the site of original injury, their persistence, and their higher rate of recurrence.[40] A higher incidence of keloids is seen in Asian and black patients.[41] The carbon dioxide laser has been widely used in the continuous wave mode for the excision of keloids.[42] Early data showed promising results for prevention of recurrence, but most long-term studies do not show a significant advantage in the prevention of recurrence by laser

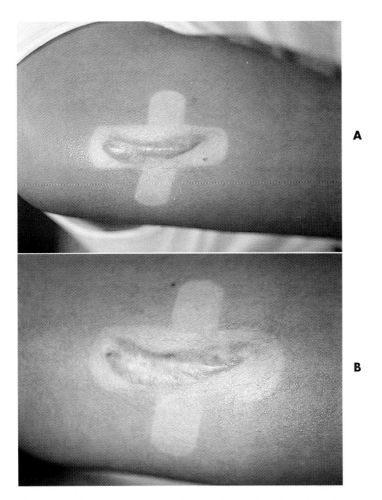

Figure 23-4   Response of a mature hypertrophic scar in a Hispanic patient after two sessions with the 585-nm flash-lamp pumped pulse dye laser.

modalities.[43] Advantages of laser excision include simultaneous hemostasis and the ligation of lymphatics, allowing for reduced postoperative edema, more precise control over depth of injury, and possible inhibition of fibroblast proliferation.[44] Adjuvant therapy with the flash-lamp pumped pulse dye laser after carbon dioxide laser excision is being investigated for prevention of recurrence.[45] Postoperative treatment with intralesional steroids, pressure, and topical silicone dressings may also prevent recurrence. As with pulsed carbon dioxide lasers, laser-treated keloid skin (if allowed to heal with second intention) will show signs of hypopigmentation (Figure 23-5).

Low-fluence flash-lamp pumped pulse dye lasers have shown some improvement in the treatment of early and mature striae.[46] Additional studies are underway to determine the efficacy of the FPDL for striae, a type of dermal scar. In darker skin types, FPDL treatment of striae can result in unacceptable hyperpigmentation and is therefore not recommended at this time. Additional wavelengths such as 532 nm at low fluences are being investigated in the treatment of striae.

Low-fluence flash-lamp pumped pulse dye lasers have shown some improvement in the treatment of early and mature striae.

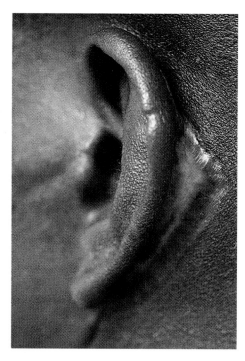

Figure 23-5   Hypopigmentation in an black patient after carbon dioxide laser excision of a keloid with second intention healing.

Hair Removal

One of the most exciting prospects for laser therapy is laser-assisted hair removal to remove unwanted hair. Several pilot studies and early data are now available with a variety of systems. A modified Q-switched Nd:YAG laser system used in conjunction with a topical suspension has been studied for hair removal.[47] Theoretically, the topical suspension is absorbed by the hair follicle, which is sensed as a "tattoo" by the Q-switched laser and then selectively destroyed. Although a slowing of hair growth may be achieved with this system, permanent hair removal is not seen. Adjustments of the pulse durations of the Q-switched alexandrite and Q-switched ruby lasers have been developed to avoid the use of a topical suspension. Early data on a long-pulsed ruby laser has shown good results in Fitzpatrick skin types I to III.[48] In darker skin, this system carries a risk of hypopigmentation. A long-pulsed alexandrite system may overcome some of these limitations, but still carries a risk of hypopigmentation. Studies without topical suspension with the Q-switched Nd:YAG laser for hair removal are being conducted. The long-term efficacy of all of these hair-removal systems need to be established.

SUMMARY

The field of cutaneous laser surgery has evolved considerably over the last few years with the development of highly selective laser delivery systems to treat a variety of skin conditions that were previously impossible to treat without significant morbidity. However, the majority of these lasers have been successful in Fitzpatrick skin types I to III. Laser treatment in pigmented skin poses significant challenges because of interference with melanin, a chromophore that is highly absorbed by most laser delivery systems. Lasers with longer wavelengths, such as the Q-switched Nd:YAG laser, have the lowest risk of pigmentary changes. When treating a pigmented individual with any laser, a conservative approach is best. Test sites and adequate long-term follow-up should be performed before treatment.

REFERENCES

1. Anderson RR, Parish JA: Selective photothermolysis: precise microsurgery by selective absorption of pulsed radiation, *Science* 220:524-527, 1983.
2. Fitzparick TB: The validity and practicality of sun-reactive types I through VI, *Arch Dermatol* 124(6):869-871, 1988.
3. Grekin RC et al: 510-nm pigmented lesion dye laser: its characteristics and clinical uses, *J Dermatol Surg Oncol* 19:380-387, 1993.
4. Kilmer SL et al: Treatment of epidermal pigmented lesions with the frequency-doubled Q-switched Nd:YAG laser: a controlled, single impact, dose-response multicenter trial, *Arch Dermatol* 130:1515-1519, 1994.
5. Dinehart SM, Waner M, Flock S: The copper vapor laser for treatment of cutaneous vascular and pigmented lesions, *J Dermatol Surg Oncol* 19:370-375, 1993.
6. Ashinoff R, Geronemus RG: Q-switched ruby laser treatment of benign epidermal pigmented lesions (abstract), *Lasers Surg Med* 12(suppl 4):73, 1992.
7. Goldman M, Fitzpatrick RE: Treatment of pigmented lesions. In *Cutaneous laser surgery: the art and science of selective photothermolysis*, St Louis, 1994, Mosby.
8. Ashinoff R, Geronemus RG: Q-switched ruby laser treatment of labial lentigos, *J Am Acad Dermatol* 27(5, part 2):809-11, 1992.
9. Sanchez NP et al: Melasma: a clinical, light microscopic, ultrastructural and immunofluorescence study, *J Am Acad Dermatol* 4:698-710, 1981.
10. Grekin RC et al: 510 nm pigmented lesion dye laser: its characteristics and clinical uses, *J Dermatol Surg Oncol* 19:380, 1993.
11. Taylor CR, Anderson RR: Ineffective treatment of refractory melasma and post-inflammatory hyperpigmentation by the Q-switched ruby laser, *J Dermatol Surg Oncol* 20(9):592-597, 1994.
12. Nelson JS: Epidermal melanosis secondary to post-traumatic hyperpigmentation. In Apfelberg DB, ed: *Atlas of cutaneous surgery*, New York, 1992, Raven Press.
13. Lowe NJ et al: Infraorbital pigmented skin: preliminary observations of laser therapy, *Dermatol Surg* 21(9):767-770, 1995.
14. Sherman R, Rosenfeld H: Experience with the Nd:YAG laser in the treatment of keloid scars, *Ann Plastic Surg* 21:231-235, 1988.
15. Kudo S, Irao R: Nevus of Ota. In Nishiyama S, Shiamo S, Hori Y: *Current treatment of skin diseases*, Tokyo, 1987, Nankado.
16. Ihm Chull-won: Nevus of Ota and nevus of Ito. In Demis DJ, ed: *Clinical dermatology*, Philadelphia, 1992, JB Lippincott.
17. Algton TS, Williams CM: Treatment of nevus of Ota by the Q-switched alexandrite laser, *Dermatol Surg* 21(7):592-596, 1995.
18. Chang CJ, Nelson JS, Achauer BM: Q-switched ruby laser treatment of oculodermal melanosis (nevus of Ota), *Plast Reconstr Surg* 98(5):784-790, 1996.
19. Taylor CR et al: Treatment of Nevus of Ota with the Q-switched ruby laser, *J Am Acad Dermatol* 130:1508-1514, 1994.
20. Fitzpatrick RE, Goldman MP: Tattoo removal using the alexandrite laser, *Arch Dermatol* 130:1508-1514, 1994.
21. Kilmer SL, Anderson RR: Clinical use of the Q-switched ruby and the Q-switched Nd:YAG (1064 nm) lasers for treatment of tattoos, *J Dermatol Surg Oncol* 19:330-338, 1993.
22. Stafford TJ et al: Removal of colored tattoos with the Q-switched alexandrite laser, *Plast Reconstr Surg* 95:313-320, 1995.
23. Anderson RR et al: Cosmetic tattoo ink darkening: a complication of Q-switched and pulsed-laser treatment, *Arch Dermatol* 8:1010, 1993.

24. Jones A: The Q-switched Nd:YAG laser effectively treats tattoos in darkly pigmented skin, *Lasers Surg Med* 1997 in press.

25. Renfro L, Geronemus RG: Lack of efficacy of the Q-switched ruby laser in the treatment of vitiligo, *Arch Dermatol* 128(2):277-278, 1992.

26. Narukar V, Vidimos AV: Lasers and incoherent light sources—new applications, *Cosmetic Dermatol* 9(6):15-17, 1996.

27. Tan OT, Murray S, Kuran AK: Action spectrum of vascular specific injury using pulsed irradiation, *J Invest Dermatol* 92:868-871, 1989.

28. Kaura AN et al: Long-pulse, high energy pulsed dye laser in treatment of port–wine stains and hemangiomas, *Lasers Surg Med* 1997 in press.

29. Tan OT, Kerschmann R, Parrish JA: The effect of epidermal pigmentation of selective cutaneous vascular effects of pulsed laser, *Lasers Surg Med* 4:365-374, 1985.

30. Ashinoff R, Geronemus RG: Treatment of a port wine stain in a black patient with the pulsed dye laser, *J Dermatol Surg Oncol* 8(2):147-148, 1992.

31. Garden JM, Balcus AD: Treatment of leg veins with high energy pulsed dye laser, *Lasers Surg Med* 8(suppl):361, 1996.

32. Narukar V, Haas AF: The effect of a variable pulse 532 nm laser with a chilling tip on vascular lesions, work in progress, unpublished data.

33. Glassberg E et al: CO_2 laser abrasion for cosmetic and therapeutic treatment of facial actinic damage, *Cutis* 43:583-587, 1989.

34. Lowe NJ et al: Skin resurfacing with ultrapulse carbon dioxide laser: observations on 100 patients, *Dermatol Surg* 21(12):1025-1029, 1995.

35. Lask G, et al: Laser resurfacing with the Silk-Touch flash scanner for facial rhytides, *Dermatol Surg* 21(12):1021-1024, 1995.

36. Khatri K: *Comparison of Er:YAG and CO_2 lasers in wrinkle removal*, ASLMS Scientific Meeting, 1997.

37. Lowe NJ, Lask G, Griffin M: Laser skin resurfacing: Pre- and postoperative treatment guidelines, *Dermatol Surg* 21(12):1017-1019, 1995.

38. Ho C et al: Laser resurfacing in pigmented skin, *Dermatol Surg* 21(12):1035-1037, 1995.

39. Alster TS: Improvement of erythematous and hypertrophic scars by the 585-nm flashlamp pumped pulsed dye laser, *Ann Plast Surg* 32:186-190, 1994.

40. Linares HA, Larson DL: Easy differential diagnosis between hypertrophic and nonhypertrophic healing, *J Invest Dermatol* 62:514-516, 1976.

41. Murray JC, Pollack SV, Pinnell SR: Keloids: a review, *J Am Acad Dermatol* 4:461-470, 1981.

42. Kantor GR et al: Treatment of earlobe keloids with carbon dioxide laser excision: a report of 16 cases, *J Dermatol Surg Oncol* 11:1063-1067, 1985.

43. Berman B, Bicley HC: Adjunctive therapies to surgical management of keloids, *Dermatol Surg* 22(2):126-130, 1996.

44. Reid R: Physical and surgical principles governing the carbon dioxide laser surgery on the skin, *Dermatol Clin* 9:297-316, 1991.

45. Lewis AB, Alister TS: Comparison of a high-energy ultrapulse CO_2 laser singly and in combination with a 585-nm flashlamp pumped pulsed dye laser in the treatment of hypertrophic scars, *Lasers Surg Med* 8(supp):31-32, 1996.

46. McDaniel D, Ash K, Zukowsk M: Treatment of stretch marks with the 585 nm flash-lamp pumped pulsed dye laser, *Dermatol Surg* 22(4):332-337, 1996.

47. Goldberg DJ: Topical suspension assisted laser hair removal: treatment of axillary and inguinal regions, *Lasers Surg Med* 8(suppl):34, 1996.

48. Grossman MC et al: Damage to hair follicles by "normal-mode" ruby laser pulses, *J Am Acad Dermatol* 35(6):889-894, 1996.

Chapter 24

Medical Therapy

Gary M. White

T he treatment of darker-skinned patients with skin conditions is similar to that in white patients, with just a few exceptions. Because pigmentation is of key importance, bleaching creams are of prime importance. Also, any topical therapy that can alter pigmentation needs to be used with caution. Finally, UVB and PUVA therapy require modifications when used on dark skin.

TOPICAL STEROIDS

Corticosteroids are capable of lightening dark skin. Less potent steroids (e.g., Classes VII, VI, and V) rarely cause hypopigmentation. In contrast, Classes I and II corticosteroids can depigment normal skin within several weeks. Figure 24-1 shows the arm of a young boy whose nummular eczema improved with betamethasone valerate, but the surrounding skin became hypopigmented. (Note also the postinflammatory hyperpigmentation.) Thus some caution must be exercised in using these agents in the darker-skinner patient. Luckily, if the potent topical steroid is removed promptly, the color usually returns to normal.

Corticosteroids are capable of lightening dark skin. Class I and II corticosteroids can depigment normal skin within several weeks.

Intralesional corticosteroid therapy, both intradermal and intraarticular, can cause hypopigmentation.[1] It may occur where injected (Figure 24-2), or it may occur more proximally in a linear fashion following the lymphatic drainage. Hypopigmentation may occur after only one treatment or after multiple injections. The lightening may take weeks or months to develop. Atrophy may or may not be seen. How intraarticular corticosteroids cause epidermal hypopigmentation is unknown. It seems likely that leakage into surrounding tissue occurs. This may originate from the joint or from the lymphatic drainage.[2] Repigmentation usually occurs, but lesions have persisted for a year or more.

CRYOTHERAPY

Cryotherapy can easily cause hypopigmentation or complete depigmentation in the darker-skinned patient and should be avoided (Figure 24-3).

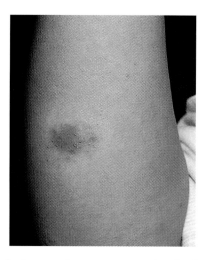

Figure 24-1   This patient had nummular eczema treated with a high-potency topical steroid. Note the central postinflammatory hyperpigmentation surrounded by steroid induced postinflammatory hypopigmentation.

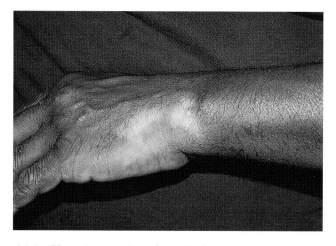

Figure 24-2   Hypopigmentation after articular injection of a corticosteroid.

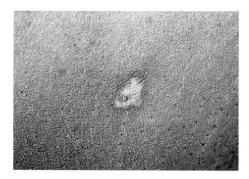

Figure 24-3   Complete loss of pigmentation after cryosurgery for a skin tag.

PHOTOTHERAPY AND PHOTOCHEMOTHERAPY

Phototherapy (UVB) and photochemotherapy (PUVA) are very valuable in the treatment of a wide variety of skin conditions. Over multiple treatments (e.g., 10 to 30), the dose of light is increased until a therapeutic benefit is achieved. The key question for each patient is how rapid can the dose be increased without burning the skin? Increasing too slowly delays benefit to the patient; increasing too quickly burns the skin. As a first approximation, the same protocol of gradually increasing exposure may be used on patients of all skin types. This approach tends to err on the side of too little light, thus delaying benefit to the darker-skinned patients. To tailor therapy to individual patients, skin typing (See Box 23-1) has been used to determine minimal erythema dose (MED) (for UVB) and minimal phototoxic dose (MPD) (for PUVA). Thus an accelerated treatment schedule can be given to the darker-skinned patients. Unfortunately, skin typing is somewhat of a crude measure of the MED or MPD because there is wide variation within a given skin type.[3]

Other more sophisticated approaches have been recommended. Carabott and Hawk[4] did weekly testing to determine the MPD. This allowed for maximal acceleration of therapy for each patient. The drawback is that weekly phototesting is needed. Bech-Thomsen, Angelo, and Wulf[5] used skin reflectance (which uses a noninvasive device to determine skin redness and pigment) to determine skin pigmentation and found it to predict well MPDs and MEDs. According to the authors, this approach could easily be incorporated into both phototherapy and photochemotherapy, resulting in more effective therapy.

Clearly, more research needs to done in this area to determine the optimal protocol for darker-skinned patients. Furthermore, those studies need to include skin types V and VI because the bulk of studies to date have focused on patients with skin types I through IV.

REFERENCES

1. Friedman SJ, Butler DF, Pittelkow MR: Perilesional linear atrophy and hypopigmentation after intralesional corticosteroid therapy, *J Am Acad Dermatol* 19:537-541, 1988.
2. Kikuchi I, Horikawa S: Perilymphatic atrophy of the skin, *Arch Dermatol* 111:795-796, 1975.
3. Stern RS, Momtaz K: Skin typing for assessment of skin cancer risk and acute response to UV-B and oral methoxsalen photochemotherapy, *Arch Dermatol* 120:869-873, 1984.
4. Carabott FM, Hawk JLM: A modified dosage schedule for increased efficiency in PUVA treatment of psoriasis, *Clin Exp Dermatol* 14:337-340, 1989.
5. Beck-Thomsen N, Angelo HR, Wulf HC: Skin pigmentation as a predictor of minimal phototoxic dose after oral methoxsalen, *Arch Dermatol* 130:464-468, 1994.

Index

A

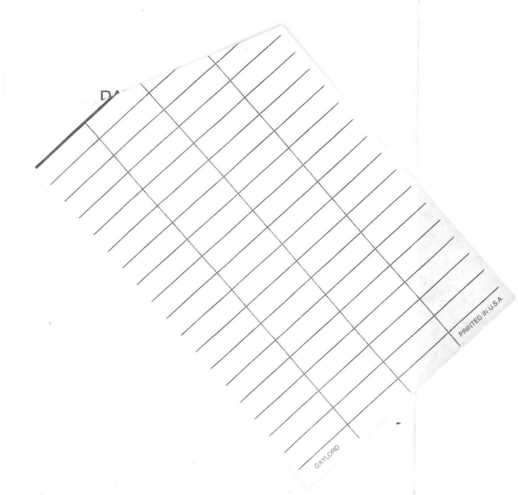

DATE

GAYLORD

PRINTED IN U.S.A.